WHY WE AGE

Solving the puzzle of aging

A STORY OF CHROMOSOMES, GENES, FATS & INFLAMMATION

Dr. Judy Ford

First published in Australia in 2019

By Expert Genetic Services

Unit 109/6 Jersey Place, Cromer NSW Australia 2099

Updated December, Copyright © Judy Ford, 2019

National Library of Australia Cataloguing-in-Publication data

Ford, Judy, 1946 -

ISBN: 9781674558936

About the Author

Judy Ford grew up in Sydney and studied Science at the University of Sydney. She obtained a first-class honors degree in Biology/Genetics in 1967 and a PhD in 1971. Her post-doctoral work in Embryology then 25 years in clinical cytogenetics motivated her research into the mechanisms of aging. She initially mostly grappled with the question of why women's reproductive potential declined so rapidly in their late thirties, especially from about 37? Then, discovering that this was a whole body 'problem' she started looking at whole body physiology.

Because of the complexity of biology and medicine, people tend to become experts in one field. It is difficult to transcend fields and link (and make sense) of cross-disciplinary knowledge. But Judy has achieved this and used her knowledge of genetics, cell biology, physiology, biochemistry and public health to make sense of the disparate research in aging. Several of her own research publications are referred to in this book.

After spending the last 12 years as a University lecturer in Postgraduate Education, Judy is now enjoying being semi-retired and writing and speaking on the research topics that most inspire her.

FORWARD

Professor Guy M Robinson

University of Adelaide and University of Cambridge

Because aging is imperceptible when looking in the mirror each day, we may be shocked when we open the photograph album and see changes across a lifetime. We can observe obvious superficial signs of aging, but what exactly is the aging process? What is changing in our bodies to deliver the external changes that we detect? What produces the 'slowing down' and inability to do at sixty what we could at twenty?

These are the sorts of question that Dr. Judy Ford has asked and investigated throughout her career. Trained as a geneticist at the University of Sydney, as a researcher in clinical genetics and human biology, and latterly as a science educator and communicator, she has worked on different aspects of human aging, asking profound and fundamental questions about aging, often overlooked. Some of the outcomes from this lifetime of research are brought together in this fascinating book, which presents new insights and directions for future research.

In her book Judy grapples with the puzzle of aging and assesses the individual pieces of research that reveal snippets of information about how we age must be pieced together, just like a jigsaw puzzle, to deliver a more complete picture. The pieces include telomeres, mitochondria, redox (reduction–oxidation reaction), oxidative stress, glutathione and healthy diets, all of which feature in the story woven around aging by Judy Ford. She examines the biology of aging, stressing the importance of our genes, though it is how they are arranged in chromosomes, and the roles played by telomeres, fats (lipids) such as Omega 3, 6 and Omega 9 that are vital to our health.

The book also considers some of the vast literature on lifestyles and diets, considering what we should, and should not, do to reduce aging and negative age-related outcomes. This includes the positives of a Mediterranean-style diet and maintaining good levels of sulfur, iodine and zinc, the need to protect our telomeres, the types of exercise we need (including for our brain) and reducing stress.

This book challenges some commonly held assumptions around aging and what helps us to age well. Using data from sources worldwide and employing simple but effective graphics, Dr. Ford tackles vital questions such as 'is the key to aging genetic make-up, lifestyle or both?

Informative and thought-provoking, the book is written in an engaging and accessible style for scientists and lay readers alike. We should all question our dietary and lifestyle choices and be more sceptic about the casual assumptions we make about our health as we age. Judy Ford has assembled an intricate, fascinating and highly readable 'puzzle' of aging.

INTRODUCTION

Isaac Newton:

'Truth us ever to be found in simplicity and not in the multiplicity and confusion of things.'

Aging is an obvious and essential aspect of living but for many different reasons, the story of how our cells age has remained disconnected and confused. In this book, I will address the important gaps in the story and although there is always more to know and the literature expands relentlessly, I will show how the key elements fit together into a cohesive picture. I hope that by understanding this process, you can take appropriate actions to minimize some of the negative aspects of aging.

The content in this book is all based on published scientific/medical research (some is my own) and other international data. My motivation for my research started early in my life. I am the youngest of four children and because of the timing of World War 2, I am more than five years younger than my closest in age, sibling. So – for those times – my parents were quite a bit older than other children of my age (my mother was 37 and my father 41 when I was born) and my grandparents were already in their sixties. This meant, of course, that by the time I was really taking much notice of other people's health, my parents were in their fifties and their parents were in their seventies.

The two age-related conditions that were most noticeable in my grandparents were osteoarthritis in *nan* and rheumatoid arthritis and early dementia in *pa*. I have now learnt that rheumatoid arthritis is associated with a three times increased risk of dementia, possibly caused by the inflammation in the tissues. But *nan,* with osteoarthritis, who struggled around with her bad hips for the remainder of her long life, had never a hint of dementia.

Nan was such a positive person. She was mentally alert and great fun until she died 'of old age', aged 95 but she struggled a great deal with her arthritis, and it was sad to see her so limited by this and in pain – though she never said so.

As a child I always wanted to know 'why' and 'how' and was never satisfied with trite answers. I decided at about age seven that I was going to be a scientist and my earlies goals were to discover the answers to important questions that were related to inheritance and biology.

When I started at the University of Sydney in 1963 aged 16, I knew I wanted to be a scientist, but I really didn't know any more than that. My career has been very influenced by serendipity but possibly because my work didn't lead me in a straight line, I have had considerable cross-disciplinary experience, and this has led to me making some very important insights that contribute to an understanding of the biology of aging.

This book, then, mainly refers to the work of the international community of scientists and data published by international organizations but here and there, I have included references to my own work when it is warranted.

My nan and pa, and my parents all led happy lives, and whilst they would certainly have benefited from some of the more recent pharmaceutical discoveries and surgical techniques, they probably would also have greatly benefited from some simple lifestyle modifications that I will describe in the chapters of this book.

I hope that you will find that the information contained in these pages is enlightening. I believe that I have finally put together many of the pieces of the current jigsaw of research findings that often seem contradictory and confusing. Of course, there is much more work to be done but at least here you will find one, consistent explanation that makes sense and allows you to make some informed decisions about your future life and lifestyle.

With my very best wishes,

Judy

PART A: THE BIOLOGY OF AGING

Chapter one

CRIKEY I'M 40 – IS IT ALL DOWNHILL FROM HERE?

How age-related changes in female reproduction give insight into the mechanisms of whole-body aging

More than 30 years ago when I celebrated my 40th birthday, many people assured me that 'life truly begins at forty'! So, is 40 the real start of aging or is it the beginning of some pleasurable change in life? Well I think that from a biological perspective both are true. Forty is the age when our peak fertility is past. For almost everyone, male and female, our fertility has peaked in our twenties and by forty we are usually approaching infertility. For women this means that they will have more difficulty becoming pregnant whilst also having a high chance of suffering a miscarriage. But men's fertility also reduces over the same period[1] [2] and what might seem a loss has many psychological gains, especially for males.

---

[1] JH Ford, L MacCormac, J Hiller (1994) *PALS (pregnancy and lifestyle study): association between occupational and environmental exposure to chemicals and reproductive outcome.* Mutation Research 313: 153-164

[2] JH Ford, HZ Wilkin, P Thomas, C McCarthy (1996) *A 13-Year Cytogenetic Study of Spontaneous Abortion: Clinical Applications of Testing.* Australian and New Zealand journal of Obstetrics and Gynaecology 36: 314-318

Middle aged men generally have far lower testosterone levels than younger men, and this usually makes them more emotionally stable and less aggressive. Females still have monthly cycles and the experience of menopause in the late forties/early fifties can be emotionally and physically stressful, but otherwise I think that the forties are generally enjoyable.

There have been various 'food fads' (or perhaps we may call at least some of them food recommendations) over the last few decades that have influenced people's weight and when I was 40, there was a strong recommendation to eat masses of carbohydrates. So, as a result of doing just that, we all gained a lot of weight. Nevertheless, many of us asked one another 'Have you put on weight, especially around your stomach, since you turned 40?' And 'yes', we all had. My mother's generation used to call it 'the middle-aged spread'!

Now in my generation this weight-gain might have been partly attributable to eating and drinking more, despite some of us exercising vigorously most days but it certainly wasn't true of my mother's generation. My mother and her peers had no 'mod cons' to help with the housework and they certainly didn't eat or drink to excess. Life, then, was quite hard physical work. So why particularly do women find that they start to put on weight at around age 40 and what has this to do with the process of aging, if anything?

How my work on reproduction first led me to investigate fats

I am going to explain how all this works in much more detail later but here I'll just tell you a little bit about my research journey that led me to find a critical connection concerning aging that is still largely ignored.

In 1972, I was employed in a research position to develop a reliable technique to discover whether a pregnant woman, aged 40 or older, was carrying a baby with trisomy 21 (Down syndrome). My work involved receiving a sample of amniotic fluid, from which I would extract cells and attempt to grow them under sterile conditions. I would then try to produce spreads of chromosomes that we could analyze under the microscope. Over the years this technique became more refined and more reliable and was generally offered to women aged 35 or older. It has since been gradually replaced with the somewhat more automated techniques that are currently available.

I had always been interested in why women in their late thirties to early 40's had this quite suddenly high risk of having a child with an extra small chromosome and this mystery became one of my key research questions over many years.

Research is generally a slow process and although most researchers make some interesting findings along the way, their individual contributions are usually small, and the big problems often remain unanswered. It's usually a case of gnawing away at the problem rather than being able to take a big bite of the apple and coming up with a solution.

But one important finding that my laboratory made was that the problem of mis-dividing chromosomes was not just confined to the reproductive cells. Rather, women of 40 and older – and others in high risk groups – also had similar errors occurring in their blood cells, when these were stimulated to divide[3].

---

[3] JH Ford, JA Russell (1985) - Differences in the error mechanisms affecting sex and autosomal chromosomes in women of different ages within the reproductive age group. American journal of human genetics 37: 973 - 983

At the time, our finding attracted worldwide media attention and not surprisingly there was a focus on the possibility of developing a blood test to measure reproductive risk. Nevertheless, although we didn't have the resources to try to research this effectively, the concept of a 'whole body' aging rather than just a 'reproductive problem' never left me.

My circumstances changed, and I had no opportunity to undertake any further laboratory research after 1996. However, in 2008 when I had funding to think and write about research on one day a week, I searched through the published research literature for any studies that might have shown one or more major physiological changes in women at about age 40. There were a few suggestive studies with insufficient (or unavailable) data but there was one large and thorough study that was extraordinarily helpful.

Perhaps strangely, the Scottish authors who had a very different focus to mine, didn't see what I saw in their results, but they were good enough to share their 'raw' data with me.
Fat metabolism and age – results of the Scottish Heart Study

The Scottish Heart study collected adipose tissue from 10,359 men and women aged between 40 and 59 years from 22 districts in Scotland. They also collected a smaller number of specimens from some younger women that although not included in their own analyses, they sent to me along with the data from the older women. So, with the help of expert statistical advice, I was able to use their *raw* data on fatty acids in females to develop a new model of changes in fatty acids with aging.

I did not receive data for the males so although it is easy to see from their published data, that a similar, but not identical, sequence of events is happening in men over this age range, my model has necessarily been developed from the female data.

I am going to explain the most important results in the coming chapters and show just how these data link to the telomere (telomerase) theory of aging but also – equally as importantly – how these data lead us to expect problems with cellular membranes. Currently, various aspects of and problems of aging are usually attributed to separate mechanisms but in fact they are all related.

This all sounds a bit complicated, but I think that once I explain it to you, you will find that it is quite easy to understand.

So, is 40 the beginning of the end?

Well, in a way 'yes' and 'yes', the middle-aged spread at least starts off as a biological change. But the good news is that there are several things you can do to stave off many of the negative age-related changes and the first of these is – as all Mediterranean's know – to have a high daily intake of extra virgin olive oil!

Chapter two

WHY FATS ARE SO IMPORTANT TO LIFE ITSELF AND YOUR HEALTH

Cells of higher organisms, their internal structure and function, and the critical roles of phospholipid membranes

The evolution of cells of higher organisms

As life has evolved, organisms have not only become more complex, but many larger organisms have permanently engulfed other smaller organisms; life then continues, and the relationship may give great benefit to both organisms. Many of the first studies of mutually beneficial or so-called symbiotic relationships were undertaken in plants where it was observed that plants such as legumes have nodules on their roots that contain *nitrogen-fixing* bacteria. These bacteria, called rhizobia, allow legumes to grow in poor soils and compete from a growth perspective with other plants. A side-benefit to us humans is that legumes can greatly replenish poor soils.

In relatively recent years, we have come to appreciate that 'we, also, are not alone'. Rather, our bodies contain a vast array of small organisms, especially bacteria that play an important role in our ongoing health. However, although this is an extremely important topic and one that we need to learn much more about, the current studies are still in the early stages and so I won't consider them in great depth in this book.

What I would like to discuss here are *organelles*. These small, functional structures within our cells, for example 'mitochondria', originally evolved from bacteria by some type of engulfment process that led to a permanent symbiotic relationship. It is important to appreciate that we don't just contain human genes and human DNA but that we are all quite a mishmash of human and lower organisms and that this creates an extremely complex situation. Nevertheless, considerable research (mostly in yeast) shows that the sub-networks within cells are fully integrated.

Thus, despite the DNA found in our mitochondria being completely different to the rest of our DNA and originating from bacteria (or similar), mitochondrial function is coordinated with the whole cellular function.

Lipids, phospholipids and fats

First to (hopefully) avoid confusion, I am going to give some definitions:

- *Lipids* are a large group of substances that are insoluble in water but are soluble in alcohol, ether, and chloroform

- *A fatty acid* is a special type of lipid called 'carboxylic acid' that has a long aliphatic chain that is either 'saturated' or 'unsaturated'. For our purposes we need to know that saturated fatty acids are generally very stable structures and unreactive whereas unsaturated fatty acids – because of their relative instability – can carry out reactions. So, generally our membranes need to contain both types of fatty acids. The saturated part will ensure that the structure is stable while the unsaturated part can play an active, functional role.

- *Phospholipids* are lipids that contain a phosphate group. They usually contain one saturated fatty acid, one unsaturated fatty acid and a phosphate group. The two fatty acids form 'tails' that are hydrophobic (water repelling) while the phosphate 'head' is hydrophilic (water attracting).

- *Essential fatty acids* are those that cannot be manufactured by our bodies and need to be consumed in our diet or by supplements BUT that does not make them more important than fatty acids that can be manufactured by our bodies!

- *Fats* are a subgroup of 'lipids' that are called triglycerides. Triglycerides (or esters) are comprised of glycerol plus three fatty acids, mostly of the types with 16, 18 or 20 carbon atoms. The composition of triglycerides is quite variable.

Cellular phospholipid membranes and their critical roles in cells

Now that you have some idea of what a phospholipid membrane is, I am going to define the most well-known of these membranes and their functions. It isn't necessary to understand the chemistry, but it is necessary to recognize the critical roles that lipid membranes play in our cells and to appreciate that saturated acids create stability but rigidity whilst unsaturated fatty acids allow flexibility and reactivity. Knowing this allows us to understand why age-related changes in fatty acid metabolism have such huge effects on our bodily functions.

1.   *Plasma membrane - a cellular boundary*

The plasma membrane is a double lipoprotein membrane that somewhat isolates the cell from its external environment. Not surprisingly, the inside layer of the plasma membrane also has connections with the internal membrane system that is called the *Endoplasmic Reticulum.* Protein tethers hold the two component plasma membranes together and these 'platforms' allow both exchange of lipids and important 'energy' signals that control cell activity.

2.   *Endoplasmic reticulum*

The **ER** or endoplasmic reticulum is an interconnected network of flattened membranes that are in fact enclosed sacs. These tube-like membranes are continuous with the outer nuclear membrane, described below. The **ER** functions both as a manufacturing and packaging system and works closely with another membrane structure known as the *Golgi apparatus,* as well as with messenger RNA and transfer RNA. The manufacturing of specific proteins uses the DNA base sequence as a template.

One of the outcomes of aging is that the **ER** processing system becomes less reliable and malfunctions can lead to misfolding of proteins. This phenomenon is commonly described as *ER stress.*

3.   *The nuclear membrane (or nuclear envelope)*

The nuclear membrane is another highly specialized double lipoprotein membrane. Its outer layer connects to the endoplasmic reticulum and its network through the cytoplasm while the inner layer interacts with the chromatin proteins that are part of the chromosomes themselves. These two membrane layers fuse wherever structures known as nuclear pore complexes are inserted.

Proteins span both parts of the nuclear membrane and consist of one group given the general name of 'nuclear envelope transmembrane proteins' (or NET for short) and lamin proteins. There are three Lamin genes, named A, B and C, that each code for a protein. Together, the three proteins create a two-dimensional matrix adjacent to the inner nuclear membrane. Heterochromatin (usually repeated sequences of DNA that have 'controlling' roles rather than 'gene-coding roles) attaches to the lamin.

A mutant form of one lamin protein (LMNA) is the cause of the *Hutchison-Gilford progeria syndrome.* This mutation that causes aging to occur from early childhood with death from about age 12, causes an abnormal distribution of chromosomes in the cells. This rare disease proves that the inner nuclear membrane proteins are critical to the spatial organization of chromosomes and that this interaction of chromosomes and the nuclear envelope is essential to normal cell division. Moreover, a large proportion of other premature aging syndromes have also been mapped to defects in nuclear lamin proteins.

Although scientists knew from electron microscopic studies in the 1970's that chromosomes often seemed to form attachments to the nuclear membrane and that the nuclear membrane was dotted with specialized pores, I don't think any of us guessed that the nuclear membrane might be an important 'player' in the regulation of cell division. In 2011, Nikolaj Zuleger and colleagues note that 'In the past 15 years our perception of nuclear envelope function has evolved perhaps nearly as much as the nuclear envelope itself evolved in the last 3 billion years!'

The details of just how the nuclear envelope organizes chromatin and chromosomes are currently under intense investigation and the roles it plays are likely to be different in mitosis and meiosis. Nevertheless, in all cells, it seems that the nuclear envelope is the tethering point for chromosomes and that in non-dividing cells of a specific type, each chromosome appears to have its own territory[4].

Some unashamed self-promotion!

In the light of the new emergence of the understanding of the importance of the nuclear membrane to spatial control, I can't help giving myself and my physicist colleague Dr Laurie Wilson a congratulatory slap on the back for our 1972 publication called 'Spatial organization of nuclear components, and the relevance to cell division', where we proposed that chromosomes had specific attachments to the nuclear membrane (at least in meiosis) that were critical to cell division!

Whilst there is consistency in chromosome positioning in some cells, there are differences between tissues and the specific positions probably relate to some activity of gene function in a tissue. Unfortunately, this area of research has been dogged by inconsistent results which I think might be caused by the selection of cells that are researched.

Many researchers choose to work on 'cell lines' because it is convenient, but most cell lines have either been derived from cancer cells or have undergone a cancerous-like transformation. Furthermore, most cell lines are grown in monolayer cultures whereas most cells grow in a three-dimensional structure that imposes many different limitations. Furthermore, whilst it is relatively easy to research cell lines, cancer and/or transformed cells, these cell types over-ride many of the rules of normal cell division and it is fool hardy to expect them to reveal the mechanisms of normal cell division.

---

[4] Ford JH & Wilson LS (1972) Spatial organization of nuclear components and the relevance to cell division. Cytobios 5, 35-42

4.   Mitochondria

Mitochondria (mitochondrion = singular) may be the most important of our organelles as they are responsible for control of ENERGY through the production of a molecule called adenosine triphosphate or ATP for short.

Mitochondria, originally derived from bacteria, have become essential elements in the cells of all higher organisms, both plant and animal. Each mitochondrion has a double layered outer membrane and a high number of extensively folded and compartmentalized internal membranes that are given the name of cristae. Mitochondria are like bacteria in size and range from about 0.75 microns to 3 microns in diameter.

Mitochondria have their own DNA, which like that of bacteria, is circular. They have 37 genes but can produce about 615 different types of protein in humans. The number of copies of DNA per mitochondrion varies between two and ten but there are no 'repetitive sequences of DNA[5]' as in nuclear DNA.

Mitochondria are 'maternally inherited'. This means that we receive all our mitochondria from our mother. When an egg is fertilized by sperm some mitochondria pass into the egg, but these are all marked for later destruction. There are some inherited diseases caused by abnormalities in mitochondrial DNA and these can only be transmitted from mother to child.

---

[5] Repetitive sequences of bases in DNA are sequences of bases that are repeated but don't have any meaning in terms of their translation to an amino acid (as usual sequences). They used to be referred to as junk DNA but are now known to have many important functions mostly related to control of protein synthesis. Repeated sequences in telomeres play a critical role in aging.

Many illnesses, and especially age-related illnesses seem to have at least *some* of their origins in mitochondria. These include Alzheimer's, Parkinson's, Stroke, Cardiovascular Disease and Diabetes Mellitus. Many studies in the last decade suggest that all these diseases involve changes in mitochondrial membranes and that the different diseases involve specific types of alterations.

5.   Lysosomes and Endosomes,

Lysosomes play a critical role in modifying cellular responses to the availability of nutrients, generalized recycling of resources and undertaking repair programs. Most of the research into lysosomes has originated from the studies of very rare genetic diseases, called by the general name of 'lysosomal storage disease'.

There are about 50 lysosomal storage diseases and they vary in severity. Many, however, are extremely serious and cause developmental delay, seizures, deafness, blindness and movement disorders.

Lysosomes carry out their functions using a very wide range of enzymes that act on different cellular chemicals using enzymatic reactions that usually require a very acidic pH that is regulated by an energy dependent pump. The lysosomal storage diseases have very serious consequences and usually involve severe degeneration of neuronal tissue in childhood.

But apart from these rare genetic illnesses, abnormal lysosomal function is also found in Parkinson's and Alzheimer's diseases and it has been claimed by some that **lysosomal *pH* control** determines cellular lifespan.

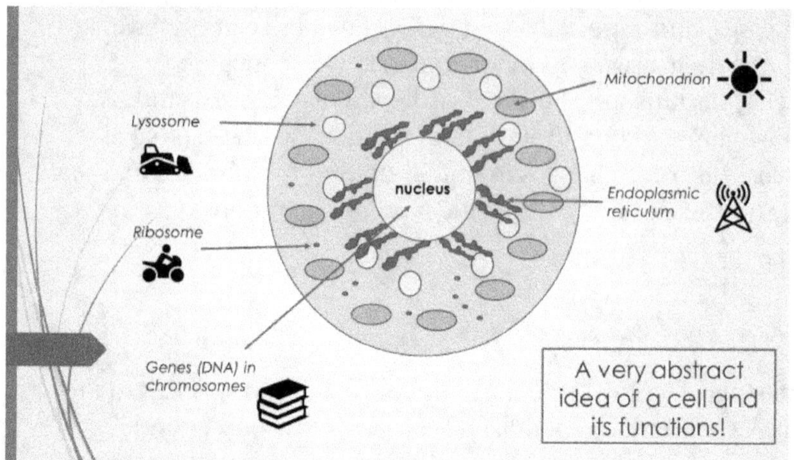

Figure: Cartoon of a cell to illustrate the functions of the components – please note that there are far more copies of everything than shown here and the arrangement is "for the convenience of the artist"!

In this cartoon it is possible to envisage a cell as being like a small village. The nucleus is the 'library', where all the information about the village is stored in genes that are organized on chromosomes. The cytoplasm is a large manufacturing center to which codes (messenger RNA) from the nucleus are transferred by ribosomes and transcribed into proteins. The many mitochondria provide energy for all the cellular functions to take place and the endoplasmic reticulum links everything together as one communication system. But, like everything else the system produces waste and the lysosomes are there as the cellular waste disposal system.

What do all these organelles have in common that might underlie age-related changes and dysfunction?

Individual cells are amazingly complex structures that perform a range of incredible manufacturing, organizational, dispersion and disposal tasks but what all the various components have in common is their **phospholipid membranes.**

Certainly, these membranes vary somewhat in their degrees of decoration, modification and specialization but at the root of all this complexity is a bi-laminate lipoprotein membrane and there is good evidence that the fatty acid composition of the cellular membranes is altered with aging. I have previously published (what I think is) a correct explanation of why and how this happens and how it relates to telomere length. Nevertheless, probably because of the complexity of aging itself, this is usually overlooked and is why I was motivated to write this book.

All the cellular organelles are very adversely affected by the age-related change in fatty acids, and while the changes in mitochondrial function might be more obvious than the changes in some of the other organelles, the decline involves all the organelles and you will see that the changes in fat metabolism occur as a direct result of cells reaching their 'telomere limit', which is the limit of their capacity to divide.

Chapter three

GENES, CHROMOSOMES, TELOMERES AND CELL DIVISION

OUR DYNAMIC GENES

What is a gene?

A gene is a 'unit of inheritance' passed on by a parent to a child (or offspring). The basics of inheritance were defined by an Augustinian monk called Gregor Mendel in the 1800's. As a gardener, he made many observations on his plants and cleverly designed experiments to test his theories. His observations have stood the test of time and even though we have now learnt a great deal about the sophistication underlying gene transmission, Mendel's findings were a critical beginning.

Every living organism uses genes as the blueprint or code that underlies its structure and functions. A single gene usually defines a single form or function. The number of genes varies greatly between small and large organisms (e.g. between fungi and elephants) but the overall composition of genes is very similar despite the huge difference in complexity of the organisms.

Genes are comprised of a chemical called DNA and each DNA molecule carries genetic information encoded within its configuration. An analogy is that DNA is rather like a book that contains information in the form of words. The arrangements of letters within the words and the words within the sentences, create the meaning. The difference is that the genetic code uses only 4 letters and each word has only 3 letters. Each 3 letter DNA 'word' or triplet is composed of three of the four bases 'adenine, guanine, cytosine or thymine' and each triplet sequence codes for a specific amino acid. The code on the DNA is directly copied by a molecule called messenger RNA that then translates the code into a sequence of amino acids, and these are then processed to create a more complex molecule known as a protein.

DNA, chromosomes and telomeres

Chromosomes are the structures in which *genes* are arranged whereas *genes* contain the coding information from which other cellular chemicals are created.

In the simplest organisms such as viruses and bacteria, their single chromosome is composed of DNA (usually) alone but in more advanced organisms, a more complex three-dimensional structure has evolved that includes proteins as well as the DNA. The involvement of protein has allowed chromosomes to become much larger, stronger physical structures that can carry many more genes, and this has been critical in the evolution of higher organisms. Each chromosome is rather like a small rope.

In 'higher organisms', the end of each chromosome has a structure known as a *telomere* that contains varying numbers of repeated specific sequences of DNA. Telomeres don't have a coding function, but they finish the ends of chromosomes neatly and prevent chromosomes from sticking to one another – as they do if any parts of the chromosomes become broken.

Telomeres are shortened as part of the process of aging, but throughout an organism's life, they have an important role of not only in defining the ends of each chromosome but in regulating many aspects of cell division.

Human chromosomes

As humans we have 46 chromosomes, a pair of each of 22 chromosomes and a special pair known as sex chromosomes. In females the two sex chromosomes are identical and known as the X-chromosomes. In males, a small chromosome known as the Y-chromosome (which creates maleness) replaces one of the X-chromosomes. This situation is reversed in birds where the males have the two X chromosomes instead!

CELL DIVISION AND CHROMOSOMES

Mitosis

There is no such thing as a typical cell, but all cells are derived from cell division and *mitosis* is the name given to the process of cell division in which two identical cells are produced from the original cell. Mitosis starts when each chromosome doubles before the two duplicates are separated into separate daughter cells.

Studies have often been undertaken on the chromosomes of cells known as fibroblasts that were initially cultured from a small specimen of skin and then grown in a monolayer in a special purpose plastic flask. Many studies of mitotic chromosomes have also been undertaken on T lymphocytes; cells taken from a sample of blood that can be very easily grown in a liquid suspension. Indeed, if you were going to have your chromosomes studied, the study would usually be done on lymphocytes grown from a small sample of blood.

To undertake a simple light microscopic study of fibroblasts, the cells can be grown on a very thin piece of glass known as a coverslip and then stained and inverted onto a glass slide for examination. On the other hand, lymphocytes (a type of white blood cell), are grown in suspension so in order to look at the cells, they need to be 'harvested' by centrifugation and then spread onto slides.

To facilitate the analysis and counting of chromosomes, in each type of preparation, cells are exposed to hypotonic (dilute) solutions, so that the cellular membranes break down and slightly disperse the chromosomes, which are then examined under a light microscope.

Light microscopy has allowed scientists to make many observations on cells and chromosomes, but electron microscopy was required to understand the different types of subcellular entities and many new types of microscopy are now being used to provide further resolution. Nevertheless, whilst the new studies add refinement, most of the well-established information in this book will have come from light and 'transmission' electron microscopy.

Meiosis

In contrast to mitosis, which occurs in all cells at some stage, meiosis is a special cell division that is only found in sexual reproduction and occurs in the ovaries (of women) and the testes (of men). During meiosis the two copies of each chromosome pair and only one copy of each chromosome passes into the special (daughter) cells that are called gametes and are known as eggs and sperm.

The process of meiosis is a little different between human males and females because whereas females have two identical sex-determining chromosomes, called the X chromosomes, males have one X and one Y chromosome. So, in male meiosis, the X and Y chromosomes form an unequal pair in order to undergo division. As you can imagine, it is very important that there is a process that ensures that each resultant sperm contains either one X or one Y chromosome! Occasionally things go wrong but not very often.

Meiosis underlies the major difference between gametes and other cells. Eggs and sperm are known collectively as gametes and the cells that generate them are called germ cells. Gametes are specialist cells that have the role of bringing *half* of the genetic material from each parent together to form a new individual with the same amount of genetic material as the parents.

Because the specialist cell division, meiosis, halves the genetic material, at the end of a meiotic cell division each normal gamete contains 23 chromosomes, one of each pair of chromosomes. Each normal egg contains 23 chromosomes and each normal sperm also contains 23 chromosomes. After a normal sperm fertilizes a normal egg, the egg then contains 46 chromosomes, exactly 23 pairs.

Mitotic Cell Division – The Critical Factor in Ageing

Mitosis is the basis of all growth, development of biological form, and ongoing maintenance of all organs and tissues. It is the way an embryo develops from an egg and how the embryo grows to be a baby and eventually an adult. It is the way our skin replaces itself and how our immune system functions. Under optimal conditions, mitosis leads to the accurate replication and separation of chromosomes such that each daughter cell is an exact replica of the parent cell and this accurate distribution of chromosomes is critical to life itself.

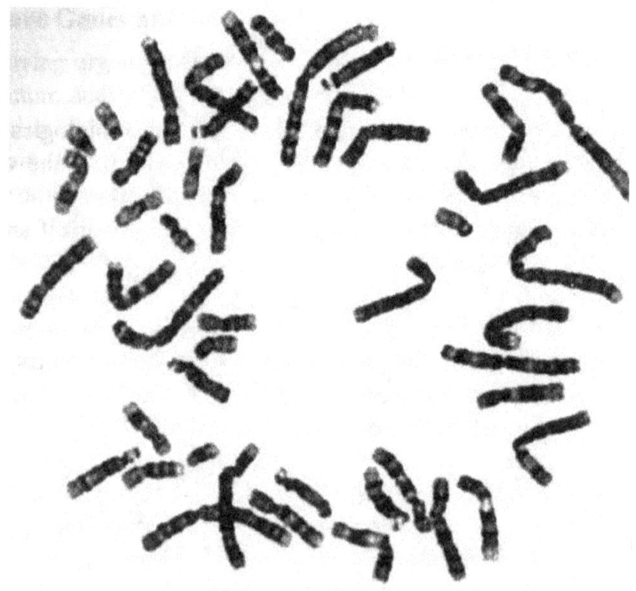

Figure: Human cell at metaphase – here chromosomes have been stained in a special way to show the individual banding profiles of the different chromosomes.

However, despite mitosis being critical to our normal existence, it is paradoxically also the function that limits our lifespan.

LIMITS TO CELL DIVISION – THE CRITICAL FACTOR IN AGEING

In 1961 Leonard Hayflick and Paul Moorhead unequivocally showed that human skin cells (fibroblasts) can only divide a limited number of times. They took biopsies of skin from people of different ages and grew them in tissue culture. Their work showed that skin cells from younger people would divide more times in culture than those from older donors but that <u>all</u> skin cells had built in obsolescence. Later it was proved that most human cells had similar limits and this observation became known as the *Hayflick Principle.*

In Hayflick's experiments, not only did the survival time reflect the limit in the number of possible cell divisions but in every case, **cell demise was preceded by less rigorous, error-prone divisions.**

Like the cell cultures, error prone divisions become more prevalent in people as they age. Cultures from older persons show a very high rate of divisional errors that result in gains and losses of chromosomes and some of these errors can cause cancer.

Since Hayflick's initial studies, further work has demonstrated other important details:

- Cells carry a 'memory' of the number of divisions they have undertaken.
- There is a rough relationship between the number of divisions cells can endure and a species' life span. Mice live for only 3 years and their skin cells have about 15 divisions compared with human skin cells that have about 60 divisions.
- The cellular clock is intrinsic to each individual cell but very similar in each cell of the same type.
- The older the person from whom cells are obtained, the less cell divisions will occur, however even very old human donors have some divisions left.
- Some normal cells are 'immortal'. They have unlimited numbers of divisions.
- The changes that induce cancer, render cancer cells immortal.
- Cells survive for some time after they have lost their ability to divide.
- Cells at birth from persons with abnormal ageing syndromes have fewer (potential) cell divisions than the cells of normal persons.

Photographs of the stages of Mitosis are shown at end of this description

Prophase is the first stage in the division process. The DNA in each chromosome has been replicated in the preceding hours and each chromosome is now composed of two chromatids that are held together at the centromere. At prophase the chromosomes seem to be somewhat randomly arranged in the nucleus, but when you look at the Figure below, you will have the impression that they are moving into new positions. The spindle is not yet fully formed.

At *prometaphase*, most of the chromosomes have moved into a ring structure and this is a sign that the spindle structure has formed and that the chromosomes are attached to it. Each chromosome is still quite long but it's easy to see that they have contracted since prophase. The two phases, prophase and prometaphase together last about 18 to 19 minutes.

At *metaphase*, the ring is fully formed, and the chromosomes contracted. The chromosomes are held in this position for about 21 minutes before the chromosome sets pull apart so there are probably some important functions occurring in the spindle at this time.

It is easy to see in the picture below that the two daughter rings are maintained as they separate from one another during *anaphase A*, which takes about 8 minutes.

The spindle then elongates during *anaphase B* and the two chromosome groups are pulled further away from one another. This process which takes about 7 minutes requires energy and this stage becomes inefficient during aging. As a result in aging cells, the <u>two chromosome groups stay closer to one another, the stage takes longer and there is more risk of various types of divisional errors</u>. A small chromosome can be noticed lagging in the upper group of chromosomes at *Anaphase B* and there appears to be a fragment remaining at the center. Such fragments can either form small micronuclei or be eliminated from both daughter cells.

In telophase, which takes about 4 minutes, nuclear membranes are formed around each of the chromosome groups and the plasma membranes start to reform between the two new cells.

In the figure below, we see the stages of mitosis as they appear in cells with minimal preparative treatment. The cells were not (as is usual) treated with colchicine in order to arrest the cells in division nor were they treated with a hypotonic solution in order to spread the chromosomes. Colchicine and hypotonic solutions destroy the ring structure of the spindle, which can be seen here quite clearly. My research team and I published the details of this technique some time ago together with some of its special applications[6]. It is thought that although the whole cell cycle takes about 24 hours, the mitotic division takes about one hour in these cells.

[6] Ford JH (2013) Protraction of anaphase B in lymphocyte mitosis with ageing: Possible contribution to age-related cancer risk. Mutagenesis 28: 307-314

Mitosis – Human Lymphocytes

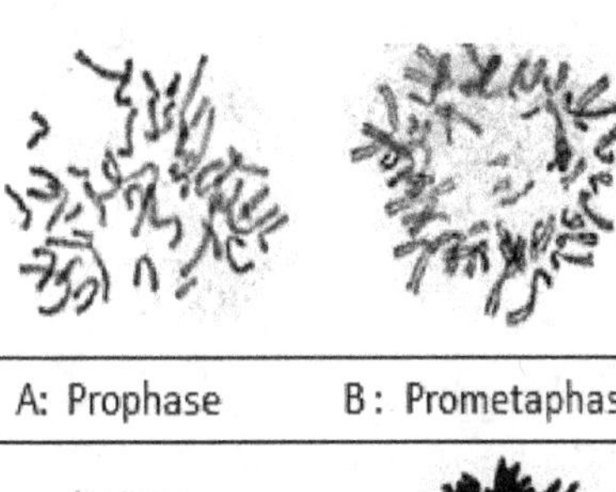

A: Prophase   B: Prometaphase

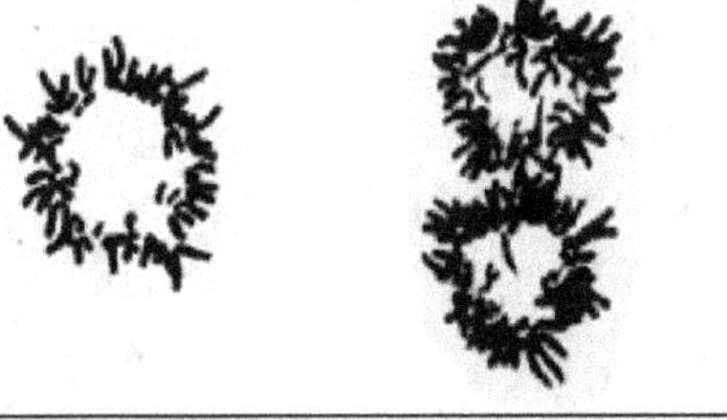

C: Metaphase   D: early Anaphase

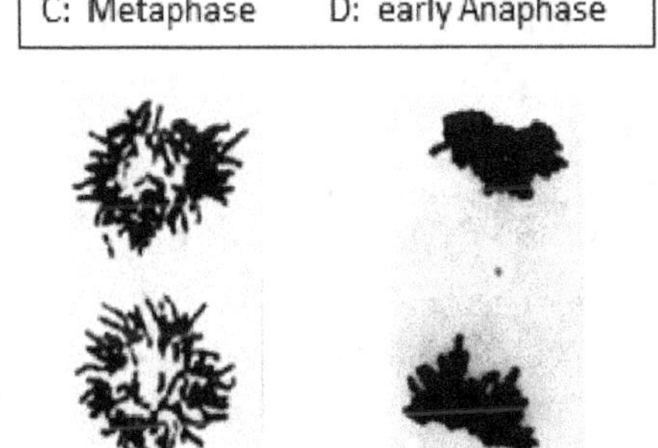

E: Anaphase B   F: early Telophase

Telomere Length controls the Capacity for Division

Research in the 1980's showed that the telomeres, the ends of chromosomes, had a special structure that is a single stranded, repeated sequence of DNA bases TTAGGG (thymine, thymine adenine, guanine, guanine, guanine) that are repeated approximately 2,500 times. Each time a cell divides, telomeres are reduced in size and this is probably because the DNA polymerase (the enzyme replicating DNA) is only able to work with double stranded DNA and the small excess 'cap' is chopped off.

Telomeres have several different roles. One is to protect the genes within the chromosomes, but another is almost certainly to give stability to the chromosome and probably also to establish its position within the cell nucleus. When chromosomes break, the broken ends can translocate within the same or between different chromosomes. Such rearrangements lead to a myriad of genetic problems (many of which are involved in congenital abnormalities and in the initiation of cancer) and an American Barbara McClintock, who studied genetic 'transposition' in maize in 1927, received a Noble prize in 1983 for her remarkable work.

Several decades later, an Australian-born scientist Elizabeth Blackburn showed that the DNA sequences that comprised the telomeres were regenerated by a special enzyme that she called *telomerase*. BUT *telomerase* is **absent** in most normal dividing cells and only **present** in germ cells, some specialized cells and cancer cells. In other words, *cell immortality* requires *telomerase* and without it, most cells have built in obsolescence. Blackburn received a Noble Prize for her work in 2009.

Once these keys to the telomere puzzle were found, research has progressed more rapidly. It was soon demonstrated that in normal cells, telomere length was reduced by EACH cell division and that in *most* cells the telomeres are not regenerated. Thus, the more cell divisions that a cell lineage has undergone, the shorter are the telomeres of the resultant daughter cells. There is a critical minimal size below which a telomere cannot function appropriately, known as *the telomere limit,* at which limit, cell division is arrested. The shortening of the telomeres ultimately limits the ability of the cells to divide.

The research about individual differences in telomere length and discussion about lifestyle and telomeres is outlined in a later chapter. For now, it is just important to know that:

1. When a cell reaches its *telomere limit* it has reached the end of its normal function.
2. On reaching its telomere limit, a cell either becomes senescent or it is destroyed by a process known as apoptosis.
3. Some stressors will initiate senescence prematurely in some cells.

Chapter four

THE TELOMERE LIMIT AND ACTIVATION OF THE P53 GENE

THE P53 GENE AND ITS ACTIVATION AT THE TELOMERE LIMIT

The *p53 gene* is found in all multicellular animals. There is sound evidence that cells have only a limited capacity to divide and that this capacity is determined by the integrity of the telomeres. Furthermore, it is well established that when the telomere limit is reached, the **p53 gene** is activated.

The p53 gene can also be activated prior to the telomere limit being reached (called premature senescence) if cellular conditions are under '*genotoxic stress*', especially due to DNA damage of some kind.

The p53 gene is often referred to as a 'cancer suppressor' gene because of the important role it plays in preventing cancer. However it also plays a major role in regulating the cell cycle and is the *master controller* of many biochemical systems.

Here are a couple of definitions of this extremely important gene:

From: Dictionary.com *"p53 gene. A **gene** that is thought to play a role in regulating cell death or apoptosis, in suppressing tumors, in regulating the cell cycle, and in stopping the cell from dividing when the DNA is damaged".*

From http://www.whatisbiotechnology.org: *"p53, also known as a tumor suppressor protein, is a gene that codes for a protein found in the nucleus of all cells in the body that helps regulate normal cell growth and multiplication. It also plays a critical role in suppressing tumors by inhibiting the division and growth of cells whose DNA has been damaged. Over half of all cancers are caused by a missing or damaged p53 gene. .... In addition to its association with cancer, p53 has recently been found to have a much broader function. Recent work has shown p53 to play an important role in in female fertility, development, stem cell division and the process of ageing."*

New insight: because *p53* regulates lipid metabolism, it has major significance in aging

When I first analyzed the age-related changes in lipid metabolism from data that was generously shared with me from the Scottish Heart study[7], I knew nothing at all about lipids.

The data I was given was a large spreadsheet that included the (de-identified) results of the laboratory analysis of fatty acids for 2,237 women aged between 20 and 65. The numbers of subjects at the lower and upper few years were low but for each other age there were 20 or more subjects. The anonymous ID for each woman, her age, her menopausal status and the values from the analysis of 12 fatty acids was included.

I started off, as I think most people would, by plotting the results of the values of each individual fatty acid against age and found that most of the fatty acids showed changes that were associated with aging. I then showed the data to a statistician who said that because there were so many correlations in the data, it should be analyzed by a technique called '*Principle component analysis*'.

This statistical technique detects the underlying patterns in data and identifies the elements that are most important. In this case, the analysis showed four major components and in three of them, there was one or more fatty acids with high positive values and one or more fatty acids with high negative values. So, at the time, not knowing anything about lipid metabolism I transcribed into 'Google' the names of the fatty acids with high positive and negative values for each factor and was thrilled to discover that each factor represented one of the key omega fatty acid pathways!

[7] I referred to this briefly in Chapter one and will describe it in more detail in the next chapter.

(I am telling you this to show you that although I had no preconceived ideas about this, the analysis revealed the critical patterns. Moreover the 'correlations' were so high that the statistician was 'amazed that biological data could reveal such clear results').

The data clearly showed that the individual components represented the three different lipid groups (so-called omega 9, 6 and 3 fatty acids) and that each of these pathways was affected by aging[8]. So, armed with this knowledge I then started to look for a way of explaining these changes in the light of what was already known about aging.

The concept of the telomere limit was well established, and it was also quite well known that the p53 gene was activated once this limit was reached. What wasn't well-known, although there were already a few publications that showed this, was that activation of p53 shut down fatty acid metabolism and perhaps the most important research showed that p53 conserved this role throughout the whole of the animal kingdom.[9]

---

[8] Ford JH & Tavendale R (2010) Analysis of fatty acids in early mid-life in fertile women: Implications for reproductive decline and other chronic health problems. American J Human Biology 22: 134-136

[9] D'Erchia AM, Tullo A et al (2006) The fatty acid synthase gene is a conserved p53 family target from worm to human. Cell Cycle 5: 750-758 doi:2622

Naturally enough I was very excited when I realized that I had uncovered a link that made sense of many of the apparently disparate findings about aging, so I published my explanation in the journal Age in 2010[10] [11].

My model still stands, however, not surprisingly, research since 2010 has made further discoveries about the p53 gene in humans. It is now well established that p53 has evolved considerably over time and is no longer just one gene but a gene system that controls fat metabolism through at least three or four different biochemical pathways. Nevertheless, the enzyme *fatty acid synthase* is the key target of p53 and its role in inducing senescence in cells that reach their telomere limit (as a barrier to tumor development) is probably the one that is most relevant to aging.

The p53 gene is **ALSO** often activated in younger cells in response to **DNA** damage but it has recently been shown that in such cells, p53 shows pulses of activity whereas in 'normal' senescence, the switch remains **ON**.

Switching the gene to 'ON' has many consequences but here I will try to decipher and explain what is now known about the key roles of fatty acids in aging.

---

[10] Ford Judith H (2010) Saturated fatty acid metabolism is key link between cell division, cancer and senescence in cellular and whole organism aging. AGE 32:231-

[11] , doi: 10.1007/s11357-009-9128-x

Activating the SENESCENCE 'ON' switch

Since p53 affects several systems simultaneously, there are multiple effects from this activation. The effect on cellular fatty acids is quite profound because as well as stopping the synthesis of any new membranes, p53 also enhances fatty acid degradation, particularly of the more biochemically reactive unsaturated fatty acids. This means that the <u>saturated fatty acid</u> content of the affected cells (and all their internal membranes) increases and the membranes become both rigid and unreactive. The altered fatty acid content of the mitochondrial and lysosomal membranes reduces the effective functioning of these organelles.

Most senescent cells are arrested in the stage of cell division[12] known as G1 that would usually proceed DNA synthesis in a dividing cell. This means that the cells are large (i.e. they would have been ready to split into two cells had DNA replication occurred) and they have increased numbers of mitochondria and lysosomes. So, not only do senescent cells have more membranes and membrane-bound organelles than other cells, those membranes are somewhat defective because they contain an excess of saturated fatty acids.

Nevertheless, **UNLESS THEY ARE DESTROYED**, the senescent cells often remain metabolically active, expressing a specific range of genes that are known as *senescence associated genes*, several of which (including p53) are controlling the senescent state.

---

[12] Byun H-O et al (2015) From senescence to age-related diseases: differential mechanisms of action of senescence-associated secretory phenotypes. BMB Reports 48 (10); 549-558

When only an occasional cell in an organ or tissue reaches its telomere limit, there are no significant consequences to the tissue and that cell is usually readily eliminated by the immune system. But as a person ages, the proportion of cells reaching the telomere limit increases and unless the immune system is very active, the senescent cells start to accumulate. Then, whenever there are excess senescent cells present, a state of 'tissue inflammation' occurs and this can have profound effects on the function of surrounding cells and tissues.

Inflammation itself is a protective response that has the function of eliminating problems by clearing out damaged cells and tissues. However, if the number of senescent cells is too high, age-related diseases, including osteoarthritis, atherosclerosis, Parkinson's disease and cancer can result. And, unfortunately in chronologically aged tissues, there are unlikely to be enough 'young' cells to come to the rescue.

So cellular senescence is in some ways a case of the cure being worse than the disease since the resultant inflammation is the cause, or at least the catalyst of many age-related pathologies.

Apoptosis –

Destruction of cells that have reached their telomere limit

An alternative biochemical pathway for cells that have reached their telomere limit is controlled by the upregulation of one of three genes PUMA, NOXA or BAX. This pathway is called the apoptotic pathway and involves the complete destruction of the old cells and presumably re-cycling of all their chemical components through other phagocytic (garbage-collecting) cells. Apoptosis was considered such an important discovery that Sydney Brenner, Robert Horvitz and John Sulston were awarded the 2002 Nobel Prize for their work.

Apoptosis is an effective system and since a specific variant of a gene called FOX03, that is involved in upregulating the genes associated with apoptosis, has been found in *most centenarians of all nationalities*, we can only assume that apoptosis is the better option for cells that have reached their telomere limits.

Unfortunately, research to date hasn't revealed a way of controlling the selection of this pathway in natural ways but not too surprisingly many researchers seeking cures for various diseases, are working in this area. A recent study[13] in mice has shown that apoptosis can be induced in mice with a peptide (part of a protein) of FOX03, with very successful outcomes. So, at some stage in the future we could see a 'senescent cell directed' apoptosis-based 'healthy aging' medication available.

---

[13] Baar MP et al, 2017: Targeted apoptosis of senescent cells restores tissue homeostasis in response to chemotherapy and ageing 'in vivo' in mice.

Can there be too much apoptosis?

The answer is a definite YES! In humans and in fact in all multicellular organisms, the balance between cell division/multiplication and cell loss/apoptosis needs to be tightly regulated. In young people it is estimated that 20-30 billion cells per day are destroyed by apoptosis whereas in adults the number rises to between 50 and 70 billion!

As well as eliminating senescent cells, apoptosis also plays a critical role in destroying cancer cells so we must never underrate its importance. However, if the system gets out of control and there is excessive cell removal by apoptosis, there may be a reduction in important cells and consequent loss of function of a whole tissue or organ.

Type 1 diabetes is an example of a disease where too many critical cells in the pancreas have been destroyed by apoptosis. Excessive apoptosis is also likely to be involved in Crohn's Disease, ulcerative colitis and several other serious autoimmune diseases.

Chapter five

FATTY ACIDS AND AGING

EVIDENCE FOR CHANGES IN FATTY ACIDS WITH AGING

The Omega groups of fatty acids

If you are like me, you will probably find much of the 'media' discussion of fats and fatty acids quite confusing. I introduced the discussion of phospholipids in cellular membranes in chapter 2 but we need to look at the different groups of fatty acids in order to try to make sense of the work being undertaken and the advice, good and bad, that is coming from some of a myriad of studies.

Here is my very simple interpretation and definitions that we need to understand. I have illustrated some of the simpler concepts in the diagram below.

1. Fatty acids are important components of other compounds (mostly called esters) that are either triglycerides, phospholipids, or cholesterol esters. In the medical diagnostic world, we hear discussion about triglycerides and cholesterol but relatively little about phospholipids, despite these being the major components of all the cellular membranes.

2. Phospholipids have **two fatty acid tails** and a **phosphate head** and generally one of the fatty acids will be what is called 'saturated' and the second 'unsaturated'. Saturated fatty acids give structural stability but are unreactive whereas unsaturated fatty acids can undertake chemical reactions.

3. The way that the hydrogen atoms in the fatty acids are arranged is important to their function. All known fatty acids have what is called a *cis* configuration, which means that the two hydrogen atoms that are next to the double bond, project outwards on the same side of the chain. Double bonds are strong, and each bond fixes the conformation (or three-dimensional structure) of the chemical chain. The more double bonds that a fatty acid has, the less flexible it is so if a chain has many double bonds in the cis conformation, it will be quite inflexible and usually quite curved in shape.

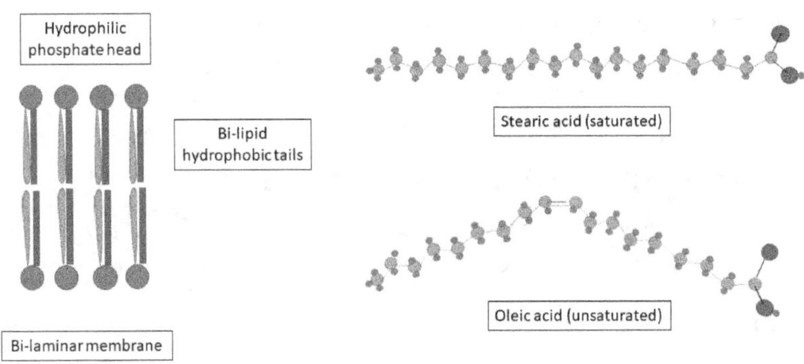

Concept of bilipid membrane structure with one unsaturated and one saturated fatty acid

In this figure – on the left we see the typical structure of a bilaminar membrane that has phosphate molecular heads (blue) on the outside and tails that are each composed of two lipids, one red (a saturated fatty acid) and the other orange (an unsaturated fatty acid). This combination gives some rigidity from the saturated fatty acid whilst still having the reactivity of the unsaturated fatty acid. On the right side of the diagram we see the difference in structure of the saturated and unsaturated fatty acids of the Omega 9 family (stearic and oleic acids, the Omega 9 (n=18) fatty acids that are the major components of our membranes. The double bond in the 9th position of the chain in the (unsaturated) Oleic acid creates a single bend.

Examples of differences in shape are found in three common fatty acids. *Oleic acid,* a short chain fatty acid, has only one double bond and only one 'kink'. By comparison, *linoleic acid,* which has two double bonds has a much more pronounced bend. Having a further double bond give *alpha linoleic acid* a hooked shape!

It is easy to understand that shapes would probably matter a great deal whenever it is necessary to create a three-dimensional structure in a restricted environment such as a membrane.

4. The nomenclature of lipids has evolved over time and there is some ambiguity. But usually 'lipid numbers' are written as C:D, where C refers to the number of carbon atoms in the molecule and D refers to the number of double bonds. This nomenclature is advised by an organization called IUPAC (International Union of Pure and Applied Chemistry).

So, for example, *stearic acid* is written 18:0 (18 carbon atoms and no double bonds) compared to *oleic acid*, which is 18:1 (18 carbon atoms and one double bond).

But there are also two further classifications, and these are ones that you will have heard in medical 'jargon'. One, like the C:D numbers describes the number of bonds. So '**saturated**' fatty acids have a straight chain with <u>no</u> double bonds. '**Monounsaturated**' have <u>one</u> double bond and hence as in OLEIC ACID above, one bend. '**Polyunsaturated**' fatty acids have more than one double bond, hence at least two bends. As a result of the extra bend, these fatty acids are more available for chemical reactions.

The second of these two further classifications uses the name '**omega groups**', which are known as 3, 6 and 9. Each group is classified according to *where* the double bond (or bend) occurs with respect to the omega (or tail) carboxyl group. Hence, in the omega 3, it is in the third position, omega 6 is in the 6th position and omega 9 (as above) is in the 9th position.

The redundancy in the classifications has arisen historically but each does serve a purpose, especially in detailed chemical analysis, despite the nomenclature being confusing. Nevertheless, we might be much further ahead in our understanding of aging if researchers had analyzed their data with respect to fatty acid metabolic pathways, rather than just referring to individual fatty acids.

Studies in middle aged humans

The Scottish Heart study whose (female) data was shared with me in 2008 was carried out between 1984 and 1986 and the published journal papers included information from men and women aged 40 to 59. A great amount of information was collected from each individual and the Dundee researchers have reported the results extensively in the biomedical literature. But in addition to questionnaire and medical data, a sample of adipose (fat) tissue was biopsied from each person's upper arm and an analysis of fatty acid composition was obtained.

It is important that you understand that the Dundee researchers published some detailed studies on the fatty acids but since they had different research interests to me, they didn't ask the same questions of the data.

Studies of fatty acids in people

In one paper[14] from the Study on fats and diet that was published in 1997, the authors analyzed results from a total of 4,357 participants (2185 men and 1929 women) aged between 40 and 59, who had both satisfactory adipose tissue samples and dietary data. **The authors reported that there were large (and highly statistically significant changes) in fatty acids that were associated with aging and were** *independent* **of diet.**

The *same fatty acids* were affected in both men and women but some of the changes were much greater in women and the concentrations of fatty acids were quite marked between the sexes.

Particularly large changes occurred in *linoleic acid* (LA) and *gamma linoleic acid* (GLA) – and for those who understand statistics the *p* value for both men and women versus age p <0.0001 – indicates a huge change. As a result of this, there is an increase in the ratio of n=6 fatty acids in the C18:2 to C18:3 groups with age, with a big decline in GLA. The researchers also found that DGLA (*dihomo-gamma-linolenic acid* C20:3, n=6) and *docosahexanoic acid* (DHA) plus *docosapentaenoic acids* (DPA) – C22:5 and C22:6, n=3) all <u>increased</u> with age.

More detailed analysis of the female data (not previously published) is shown below in Figures a to d.

---

[14] Bolton-Smith C, Woodward M & Tavendale R (1997) Evidence for age-related differences in the fatty acid composition of human adipose tissue, independent of diet. European J of Clin Nutrition, 51: 619-624

Because the Scottish research group was kind enough to share their original (female) data with me, I have been able to create the following four graphs to show just how impressive the data is. These results depicted are from the 'Factor analysis' (Principal component analysis) and do not represent the actual values of the individual fatty acids. Moreover, it is necessary to understand that in most analyses of these types of tissues, all laboratories are confined to measuring *proportions* e.g. the amount of x in a sample of size y, so a change in one component will almost inevitably cause a change in another.

The statistical analysis identified the activity of the fatty acids in the three key *omega* groups (omega 3, 6 and 9) as independent factors but the 18:3 *gamma-linoleic acid* was also identified as being an independent factor. This might reflect the fact that the omega 3 and the omega 6 pathways share enzymes that preferentially desaturate the omega 3 pathway because it is the more important.

All these changes in fatty acid metabolism *start* at about age 40 and this coincides with the age at which there are very significant changes in reproduction.

Ages at which we observe specific changes in women

From age 40 onwards, with remarkably little variation, we observe a large and continuous <u>increase</u> in the proportion of the very long chain omega 3 fatty acids (Figure b) of the type we find in fish oil, and we also see a massive drop in all the omega 6 fatty acids from the same age. *Linoleic acid, gamma linoleic acid, eisosenoic* and *arachidonic acids* are all decreased at about the same rate and this is probably explained by a continuous age-induced reduction in the activity of the enzyme known as delta-5-desaturase. **The omega-5 and omega-6 pathways are both desaturated by this enzyme and if it is limited, then it will preferentially desaturate the omega-3 pathway at the expense of the omega-6.**

Changes in Omega 9 Fatty Acids with Age

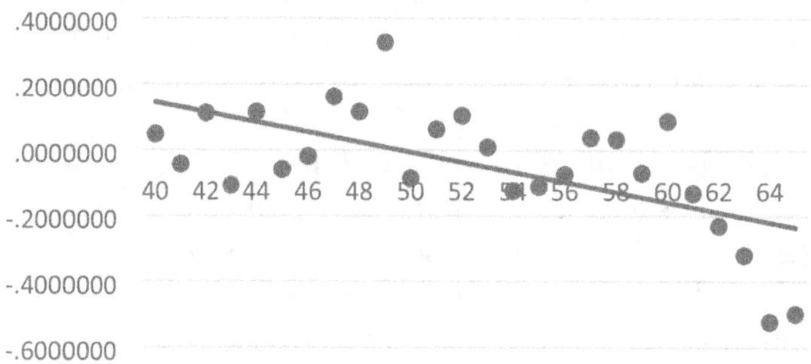

Figure a: Reduced function of CoA desaturase-1 (= Delta 9 desaturase) results in lowered 18:1 oleic acid. The ages are shown across the middle and are a little hard to see but the age starts at 40 and goes to 64. You can see a gradual decline from 40 to 60 and then a more rapid decrease from 60 to 64.

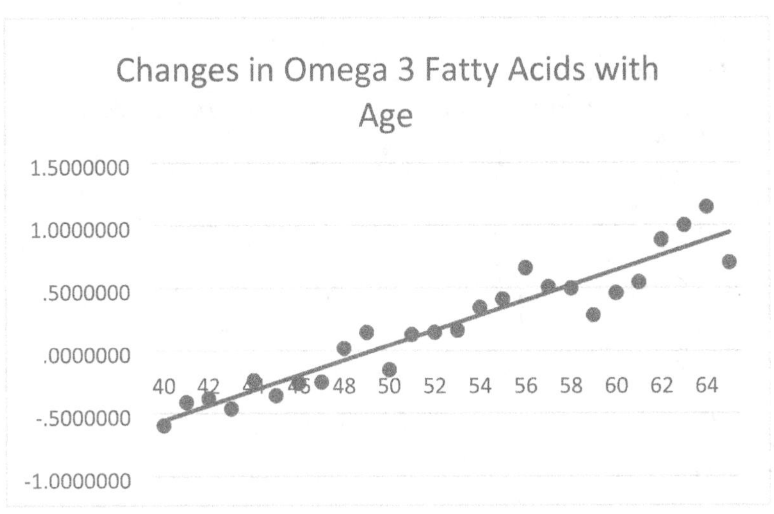

Figure b: Reduced function of Delta 5-desaturase with age. Arachidonic acid is low when compared to the long chain Omega 3 fats – the enzyme preferentially desaturates omega 3 fats if they are present – so they rise, relative to other fatty acids.

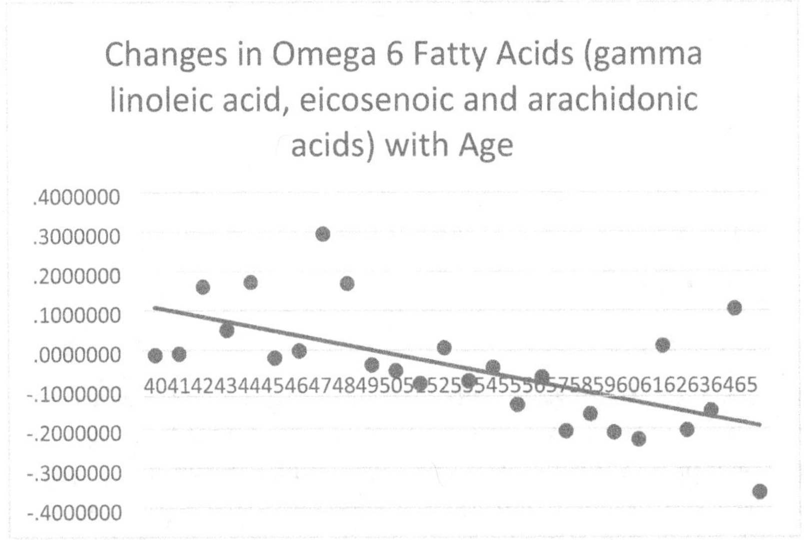

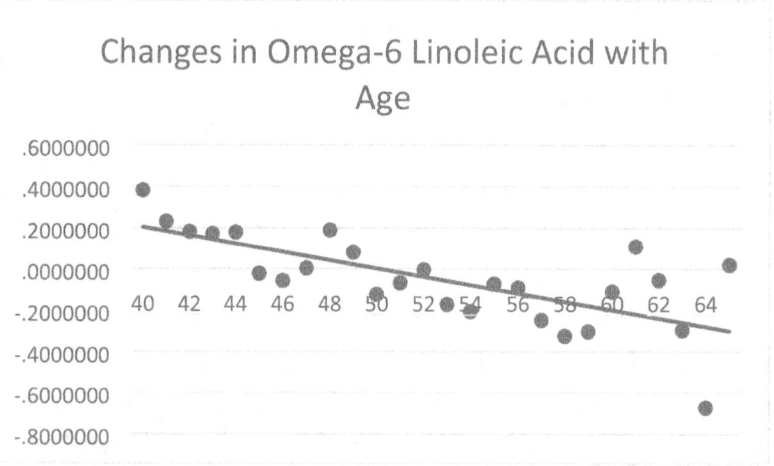

Figure d: Only the omega 6 fatty acid, 18:2 linoleic acid contributes to this factor and like the other omega 6 fatty acids, its levels decline with age.

Supportive data

The data presented in the graphs above clearly shows that there are dramatic changes in the fatty acid composition of *adipose tissue* that occur with age, but it is essential to show that similar results are found in other studies that examine fatty acids and aging. It is also important to discover whether the changes are also found in other tissues.

There is no equivalent data to the Scottish Heart Study, but below are two other sets of data that show similar types of results – i.e. that the conversion of saturated fatty acids to unsaturated fatty acids is inhibited by aging.

The next set of data was obtained from the brains of mice and this is helpful if you know how mouse ages equate to human age! The Jackson Laboratory, who are major mouse breeders estimate that a mouse aged 3 months is equal to about an 18-year old human, an 8-month old mouse to about a thirty-year old and a 26-month old mouse is equal to a human aged about 75. So, here it is easy to see in the Table below that the ratio of 18:1/18:0 greatly declines in old mice just as it does in humans although the conversion of 16:1/16:0 is not as affected.

Fatty acid (weight) ratio	Age 3 months	Age 8 months	Age 26 months
16:1/16:0	0.194	0.103	0.106
18:1/18:0	0.899	0.916	0.028

Table: Fatty acids in brain lipids of mice of different ages[15]
Conversion of stearic to oleic acid is greatly inhibited in the old mice.

Oleic acid (18:1) was also found to be reduced in the membranes of blood erythrocytes (red blood cells) in studies of cognitive decline in humans. In this study, it is easy to see that the average levels of stearic acid are increased, and oleic acid decreased in the membranes of people with cognitive decline.

---

[15] Horrocks LA et al (1975) Changes in brain lipids during aging. Neurobiology of Aging 16: 359-367

Fatty acids (% of total FA)	No cognitive decline (n = 219)	Cognitive decline (n=27)
Stearic (18:0)	13.06	13.53
Oleic (18:1)	11.07	10.93
Ratio	0.848	0.808

Table: Fatty acids in red blood cells in normal people and those with cognitive decline[16].

These data were obtained from the EVA study – The whole study population included 1389 volunteers born between 1922 and 1932 and living in Western France. This study measured erythrocyte (red blood cell) membrane fatty acid composition in 1995 in 246 men and women aged between 63 and 74 years. Their cognitive abilities were assessed over the following four years and moderate cognitive decline was assessed as a decline of > or equal to a 2-point decrease over those years.

[16] Heude B, P Ducimetiere & C Berr (2003): Cognitive decline and fatty acid composition of erythrocyte membranes – The EVA Study. Am. J. Clin Nutr. 77: 803807

The differences seen here are not as great as those in other tissues and this almost certainly reflects the fact that red blood cells only have a life of about 120 days and are produced by a multipotent stem cell that has a greater replicative capacity than some other cells. However, the multipotent stem cells that give rise to red cells do still exhibit telomere shortening and they also seem to prefer the white cell pathways as they age.

IN SUMMARY

Analysis of the fatty acids in whole tissue (adipose = fat tissue biopsy taken from the upper arm) shows that major changes in the fatty acid composition occurs with aging. The graphs shown here are female data but the male data and results for some of the individual fatty acids can be seen in the original publications that I have referenced.

Several key fatty acids are reduced by aging, but the body tends to preserve the long chain Omega 3 fatty acids at the expense of the Omega 6 fatty acids. The fatty acids that are most affected by age are <u>Omega 9 Oleic Acid</u> (found in Olive Oil) and the <u>Omega 6 Gamma Linoleic Acid</u> (found in Evening Primrose Oil).

Chapter six

CALORIE RESTRICTION, FATTY ACIDS AND AGING

CALORIE RESTRICTION IN RODENTS: CONFIRMATION OF THE 'TELOMERE LIMIT/P53/FATTY ACID MODEL OF AGING'

What is calorie restriction?

The first study of calorie restriction (CR) was undertaken as long ago as 1935 by a group at Cornel University, led by McCay. Their results were impressive and all the studies that have been conducted since have found similar outcomes.

There have been modifications to experiments on CR but most studies to date have been undertaken in rats and mice and the experimental animals have been given a diet 30% to 60% less than usual at various times in their lives. The age when the CR is commenced, the amount of restriction and the breeds of animals used have all influenced the results but overall, CR used early in life has greater benefits than even less calorie intake commenced later in life.

Intermittent fasting (e.g. alternate day feeding) has also been found to reduce the negative effects of aging and increase lifespan in rodents however, although we have seen the adoption of the '5:2' diet and similar diets in recent years, the published human studies have had very mixed results.

Phopholipid membrane composition and CR in rats

The next two tables (next page) show how mitochondrial membrane phospholipid composition was altered by age and food restriction in Fischer 344 rats[17]. The tables show my calculations from the data presented in the paper by Laganiere & Yu (1993) as the authors did not summarize the data in this way. In these experiments, animals were either allowed to eat as much as they desired AL = ad libitum or were FR = food restricted.

These results show that CR particularly targets the Omega 9 fatty acid pathway and we will see from other data that this is probably because **CR inhibits mitosis** and thus slows the rate at which cells reach their telomere limits.

---

[17] Laganiere S & Yu BP (1993): Modulation of mitochondrial membrane phospholipid composition by age and food restriction. Gerontology **1993**;39(1):7-18.

The fatty acids in each of the two common membrane phospholipids were measured and the ratios are shown for the palmitic (16:0) to palmitoleic (16:1) and stearic (18:0) to oleic (18:1) fatty acids. The results are similar in each of the two phospholipids namely that there is a reduction in the activity of each of the pathways with aging that is expressed as <u>a reduction</u> in the ratios of the saturated to unsaturated fatty acids but the age induced change is much greater in the AL groups than the FR groups. In other words, food restriction slows down the rate of aging in rats and this affects fatty acid metabolism.

Phosphatidylcholine

Age	Six months		18 months		24 months	
Food coding	AL	FR	AL	FR	AL	FR
Ratio 16:1 to 16:0	0.044	0.046	0.045	0.047	0.021	0.037
Ratio 18:1/ 18:0	0.180	0.221	0.169	0.272	0.133	0.210

Phosphatidylethanolamine

Age	Six months		18 months		24 months	
Food coding	AL	FR	AL	FR	AL	FR
16:1/ 16:0	0.036	0.045	0.031	0.045	0.020	0.032
18:1/ 18:0	0.154	0.212	0.149	0.233	0.131	0.207

In their review called 'Aging, Adiposity and Calorie Restriction', Fontana & Klein[18][19] listed six key outcomes of CR and made the comment 'The precise biological and cellular mechanisms responsible for primary and secondary aging are not known but likely involve:' They then created their list.

However, in the light of understanding about the key effect of aging on fatty acid metabolism, I am both reordering and modifying their list. Many of the other components of the sequence they describe are direct or indirect results of the activation of *p53* and changes in the two fatty acid pathways. Most importantly I will start with alterations in fatty acid metabolism. In all these results, it is important to remember that although most studies have focused on changes in mitochondria and mitochondrial function, all the cells' phospholipid membranes and organelles are affected by the changes in fatty acid metabolism, including the liposomes[20].

On the next page I have created a sequence of the key stages of aging that occur in most of our cells but there are some cells, that are generally known as stem cells that are exceptions to this rule. Stem cells have telomerase and can thus replicate their telomeres and (possibly) never undergo senescence. There are also some blood cells that express small amounts of telomerase, probably as a repair mechanism. These are the only normal cells that express telomerase and generally when telomerase activity is acquired it is by *rogue cells* and leads to cancer.

---

[18] Fontana L & Klein S (2007) Aging, Adiposity and Calorie Restriction, JAMA 297:

[19] -994

[20] Despite the vast number of studies on (a) mitochondrial dysfunction in aging and (b) the extensive studies on diet and health, there have been few studies on membrane lipids, diet and mitochondrial physiology. Those that have been undertaken show that dietary lipids can have profound effects on mitochondrial composition and function.

In general, calorie restriction seems to work by switching off cell division and whilst this has many beneficial effects, recent research from the Leibniz Institute on Aging – Fritz Lipmann Institute, has shown that CR also restricts the number of immune cells and can compromise immunity.

Telomere & p53 sequence of events in Primary & Secondary Aging

1. p53 system is activated in cells that reach their telomere limit.

2. The key gene 'fatty acid synthase' is inactivated and this results in changes in the ratio of fatty acids, especially 18:1/18:0.

3. Activation of p53 stops lipid synthesis and lipid metabolism and this alters the chemistry of phospholipid membranes.

4. Altered membrane lipids impair the function of all cellular organelles especially mitochondria and lysosomes.

5. Mitochondrial stress causes major problems in loss of cellular energy by reducing their major function of creating ATP.

6. Mitochondria usually 'manage' reactive oxygen species. Their decreased function augments superoxide production that aging mitochondria can no longer 'manage'. This has a major role in creating inflammation.

7. Reduced function of cellular lysosomes (also initiated by changes in membrane lipids) leads to an accumulation of 'cellular waste' and this further interferes with normal cellular function.

8. The increased proportion of cells becoming senescent, with and without their efficient removal, eventually leads to a decrease in cells (including neurons and muscle cells) as well as deterioration in the structure and function of cells in all tissues and organs.

Chapter seven

CELLULAR DEFENCE SYSTEMS: IMPORTANCE OF ZINC AND SULFUR

But wait there's more!

Our complex cellular systems have been evolving over a very long time and it would be unreasonable not to expect that there would be a few other back-up mechanisms ready to protect us from the ravages of disease, illness, accident and aging.

Here is a list of five of our most important defense systems:

a)   The immune cells

b)   Superoxide dismutase enzymes

c)   Taurine (a previously ignored defender)?

d)   Glutathione S transferase

e)   The 'heat shock' *Hsp* gene family

IMMUNE SYSTEM AND CELLS

Our immune system is established during our embryonic development although some components are not active until certain stages of post-natal life. But like all other components in the body, our immune system ages and this results in:

- Greater susceptibility to infections
- Less effective responses to vaccinations

The increased prevalence of cancer seen with aging, and both autoimmune and chronic diseases are sometimes also included as deficiencies in immune function. Nevertheless, although an aging immune system will certainly provide less effective surveillance of these conditions, the diseases themselves are almost certainly induced at a greater rate than at earlier ages as a direct result of the aging process.

There are some lifestyle strategies that might reduce unnecessary 'wear and tear' on the immune system however here, I will just briefly describe the different elements of the immune system and discuss some of the specific changes that occur with aging. Nevertheless, it is essential to realize that current research into the immune system is making some surprising discoveries and since the whole field is exceptionally complex, I will only cover this in a very basic way.

Conventional analyses of blood reveal several different types of cells that fall into the general categories of:

(a) erythrocytes – red blood cells that carry oxygen around our bodies,

(b) B and T lymphocytes –both of which are involved in triggering our immune responses. Both types of lymphocytes are involved in recognizing harmful pathogens such as bacteria and viruses, but they can also recognize some other parasites as well as dead cells.

Both types of lymphocytes are initially produced by the bone marrow, but T cells migrate to the thymus gland where they complete their maturation. In contrast, B cells complete their maturation in the bone marrow itself. B lymphocytes tend to destroy pathogens through the production of antibodies on their surfaces whereas cytotoxic T cells phagocytose, i.e. they engulf and destroy pathogens. None of the cells work alone and one class of T cells called T 'helper cells' is a first-line defense cell that then activates the other types of lymphocytes.

(c) Granulocytes – this group includes several different cell types: monocytes, neutrophils, eosinophils and basophils. Of these, the neutrophils and monocytes tend to be mostly involved in killing pathogens. For example, if you cut yourself, neutrophils will rush to the scene and soon be producing pus, whereas the monocytes (rather like garbage trucks) will arrive a little later and remove all the dead cells from the scene of the accident!

Eosinophils and basophils on the other hand are often slightly over-protective and these cells are quite likely to over-react and lead to allergic reactions.

From the perspective of aging, immune cells are like all other cells. They are composed of masses of lipoprotein membranes and organelles and because the body has a limited capacity to produce new cells, as we age the proportion of senescent immune cells will increase.

But aging also affects the sophistication of the immune system. So, beyond the direct effects of aging on the number of cell divisions, aging is also associated with deterioration of the organs – namely the bone marrow and the thymus – in which the different types of blood cells undergo their maturation and differentiation.

Both the bone marrow and thymus show age-related fatty deterioration that *may or may not be amenable to improvement* through dietary lipids. To date, very little research has been undertaken in this important area.

SUPEROXIDE DISMUTASE

Superoxide dismutase is a critical antioxidant defense mechanism in nearly all living cells that are exposed to oxygen. I mentioned earlier that the age-related decrease in mitochondrial function augmented the production of superoxide radicals and that these are highly toxic and must be annihilated.

The enzyme that metabolizes superoxide in humans and most other higher organisms is called *superoxide dismutase*. There are three forms of this enzyme in humans known as *SOD1, SOD2 and SOD3*. *SOD1* is found in the cytosol or cellular fluid and *SOD3* is found in the intracellular fluids (the fluids between the cells of a tissue) and each of these enzymes is dependent on **copper** and **zinc** for their function. Both copper and zinc need to be in the diet at 'sufficient' but not excessive levels. Zinc is also important for the support of heat shock proteins as discussed below.

SOD2 is found in mitochondria and this important enzyme, which in some ways can be thought of as being at the site of critical action, is dependent on *manganese* for its action. SOD2 is sometimes referred to as *MnSOD* because of its importance as the key antioxidant in mitochondria.

....and just to emphasize the importance of the SOD enzymes, mutations in the gene for SOD1 cause familial amyotrophic lateral sclerosis (FALS), which is a form of motor neuron disease.

GLUTATHIONE-S-TRANSFERASE (AND THE NEED FOR SULFUR)

Whilst the SOD genes play critical roles in removing the superoxide radicals and are our most important antioxidants, Glutathione-S-transferase (GST) is a major detoxifier. It particularly removes substances given the general name of xenobiotics, which are toxins and include most substances that are foreign to an organism or are not part of normal nutrition. The compounds that are targeted by GST include a diverse range of environmental or otherwise exogenous toxins that include chemotherapeutic agents and other drugs, pesticides, carcinogens and variably derived 'epoxides'.

Many of the toxic substances managed by GST come from our external environment, either by ingestion or respiration, but some are generated by metabolism itself. These internally produced toxins – mostly epoxides – mostly come from the peroxidation of lipids and these are greatly increased in aging through mitochondrial dysfunction. Selenium (another trace element) is required in the synthesis of GST.

GST, aging and Sulfur

To ease some of 'the pressure' on GST, we can both try to improve the state of all our membranes by paying attention to the fatty acids in our diet, and by avoiding 'toxins', including medications (where appropriate). However, since *Glutathione-S-transferase* needs to be upregulated to cope with the increased inflammation produced by aging tissues, and the enzyme is highly dependent on the availability of sulfur, the demands for sulfur increase with aging. Cellular levels of glutathione are reduced by approximately 50% from about age 60 (see Table below) so in order to resist this decline, we need to increase our intake of dietary sulfur.

Glutathione levels in males are lower than those in females until the age of 60. Thereafter, on average, the levels in females decline faster as shown in the Table.

Sulfur is the third most abundant mineral in our bodies by weight and it has many other critical functions as well as supporting GST. As we age our need for sulfur increases so much that if our intake is insufficient, the body will set its own priorities and simply take the sulfur it needs from our cartilage tissue.

We aren't alone in this need as it applies equally to all mammals, and measurements taken from arthritic cartilage in horses show that the level of sulfur is reduced to about one third of the level of normal tissue. So insufficient dietary sulfur leads to osteoarthritis. It may also increase the risk of several other age-related illnesses.

Table: Glutathione content in human lymphocytes by age[21]		
Age Group	Subjects	GSH (nmol/mg protein)
20-40	Males (n=20)	19.4 ± 1.8
	Females (n=21)	23.8 ± 3.2
41-60	Males (n=21)	16.8 ± 1.2
	Females (n=20)	19.0 ± 1.8
61-80	Males (n=22)	13.3 ± 0.9
	Females (n=20)	11.2 ± 0.9

[21] Van Lieshout EMM & Peters WHM (1998) Age and gender dependent levels of Glutathione and Glutathione-S-transferases in human lymphocytes. Carcinogensis 19: 1873-1875

Like many of our very important genes, GST is a large family of genes that are found in plants and animals as well as in some of the microbes. The omega class called GSTOs differ from some of the other GSTs by having cysteine as part of their structure and by being extremely genetically variable. Large genetic studies have revealed that some of the GSTO genes are associated with the age of onset of several of the neurological genes of aging, namely Alzheimer's disease, Parkinson's disease as well as amyotrophic lateral sclerosis (ALS).

Of great interest is that genetic linkage studies have also found that in addition to the GSTO1 gene, the gene *stearoyl-CoA desaturase* (the Omega 9 desaturase that converts the fatty acid stearic acid to oleic acid) is the <u>second of four genes in a gene cluster</u> that strongly links to the age of onset of Alzheimer's disease.

TAURINE

Taurine is sometimes referred to as an amino acid because it is a sulfonic acid with an amino group. Because Taurine isn't involved in protein synthesis, it has largely been ignored until relatively recently. However, taurine is in fact ubiquitous and is the most abundant, free amino acid in many tissues, including the retina of the eye, the heart, brain, skeletal muscle and in white blood cells where it is found in high concentration.

Taurine has been found to have a key role for preventing oxidation-related injury and the emergence of new molecular laboratory techniques in the last decade has allowed much more research into its functions. For example, taurine metabolism is known to be reduced in diabetes and thus, when taurine was added to a cell culture study of hyperglycemia, it first reduced the generation of reactive oxygen species (ROS) by 34% and this in turn reduced the rate of cell death by apoptosis by 78%.

It is now recognized that taurine has at least three important and possibly separate roles, one as an antioxidant, a second in stabilizing energy transport chains and thirdly, taurine may be a neurotransmitter 'in its own right'. All these roles mean that it contributes to the support of your overall central nervous system. There is also growing evidence that taurine blocks (some) apoptosis and through that role may play an important role in reducing age-related disabilities. It seems to have many important roles in the health of eyes – especially of the macular - and in reducing over-reactivity of the nervous system.

In addition to these roles, taurine also has a specific role in providing a substrate for the formation of bile salts in the liver. Through its activity in the liver, taurine is reported to have a special role in increasing the mobility and fluidity of the membranes of hepatocytes (liver cells).

Dietary taurine is found in meat, fish and some algae but is also added to some 'energy' drinks and used in many different medical treatments. Athletes may particularly benefit from its roles in helping maintain hydration and electrolyte balance in cells.

So, this one, largely ignored amino acid has key roles in:

- Regulation of the function of the immune system
- Maintaining electrolyte balance and thus hydration in cells
- Formation of bile salts and maintenance of healthy liver cells
- Supporting the overall health of the nervous system

THE 'HEAT SHOCK' *HSP* GENE FAMILY AND ZINC INTAKE

Heat shock proteins were named shortly after their discovery in the Drosophila fruit fly in the early 1960's, when it was observed that the gene was activated when animals were stressed by dramatic changes in temperature. The family of genes, now called HSP for short have been found in bacteria and fungi as well as higher organisms and they play a critical role in 'chaperoning' proteins. The HSP genes play this chaperoning role at *all* times of stress and this includes when cells are exposed to COLD, heavy metals, low oxygen (hypoxia), radiation, deprivation of nutrients and all other exposures to toxic stress, infections and exposure to inflammatory processes. This means, of course that they are very important during aging when cells reaching their telomere limits become senescent and inflammatory.

HSP genes play a role in cells that is somewhat like the leadership team in a sports group or prefects at a school. This is a supportive or chaperoning role that keeps all the other proteins 'in order': they make sure that the proteins are assembled and folded correctly and help correct mistakes.

When a new protein is formed by a cell, the gene known as *HSP40* checks for errors and then delivers a newly formed chain of amino acids to the gene *HSP70*. *HSP70* grabs the new molecule and helps to fold it into its proper functional form before releasing it. *HSP60*, on the other hand attracts any new amino acid chain or protein that has lost its proper structure and internalizes it. Then remarkably, chemical forces within the cage-like structure of *HSP60* reorganize the protein into its correctly folded shape!

Once all these checks and corrections have been made, another gene HSP90 receives the correctly folded proteins from the other HSP chaperones and joins them together to form a larger more complex protein structure that has some important functional role.

Immune cells can often provoke a response against cancerous or infected cells but in order to do this, the immune cells need to be alerted to the problem. HSP90 as well as another gene *HSP70* play key roles in identifying problems and alerting the immune system!

Rather like the watchdog presenting the evidence to his master, the HSP proteins deliver antigens from diseased cells to the immune system's 'antigen presenting cells' or APCs. Then after internalizing the antigen, the APC releases inflammatory signals through which other immune cells are recruited. The rogue cells can now be identified by the antigens on their surfaces and thus recognized can be killed by (so-called) killer T-cells!

The stress response appears to decline with age but perhaps this reflects the increased demands put on ALL the defense systems by SENESCENT CELL induced INFLAMMATION? Needless-to - say, supplementation with zinc boosts the stress response in older people[22] and zinc deficiency in the elderly may well be a cause of immunosenescence, including ineffective responses to vaccination.

In a later chapter I will discuss the minerals we need to support our aging cells, in more detail. For now, I have created an inset, in which I present a simplified summary of the previous inset and add the prefect and watchdog systems into the list.

---

[22] Putics A et al 2008: Zinc supplementation boosts the stress response in the elderly: Hsp70 status is linked to zinc availability in peripheral lymphocytes. Exp. Gerontology 43: 452-461

SENESCENCE: Telomeres, p53 and fatty acids
& CLEARING systems

sequence of events in Primary & Secondary Aging

1. The p53 system is activated in cells where the chromosomes reach their telomere limit

2. The key gene 'fatty acid synthase' is activated, fat metabolism is suppressed, and this leads to changes in the lipid content of ALL membranes, but the lowered content of oleic acid is especially important.

3. Alteration in lipid content impairs the function of all cellular organelles and hence SENESCENT CELLS are HIGHLY INFLAMMATORY. Reduced function of the lysosomes leads to increased 'cellular waste' and loss of mitochondrial function to decreased energy and less detoxification.

4. Immune cells decrease with age but still play critical 'clearing' roles, especially in conjunction with heat shock proteins. The system is very dependent on adequate **zinc.**

5. Superoxide dismutase (SOD) clears superoxide radicals. Reactions require **copper, zinc** and **manganese.**

6. Taurine is an antioxidant and stabilizes electron transport chains. 'Early' research results suggest it may reduce several age-related diseases.

7. Glutathione-S-transferase is a major detoxifier that is critical in healthy aging but is dependent on sulfur. If sulfur isn't readily available, it is removed from the joints and causes osteoarthritis. Increasing dietary intakes of sulfur are important for healthy aging.

PART B:
INTERNATIONAL DATA
– A CAUTIONARY TALE

Chapter eight

Key characteristics of long-living populations of people throughout the world

Is the key to successful aging: genetic make-up, lifestyle or both?

There are a few places in the world where people are renowned for having longer and healthier lives than average. Naturally, researchers have looked at these people and their lifestyles to see whether the advantage is just genetic or whether there are some lifestyle differences that might guide the rest of us? We do, however, need to be cautious whenever we decide to adopt only parts of a culture because there are often critical components that are missed, and others can easily be taken out of context.

First, in order to characterize these populations, they need to be isolated. There is restricted migration both in and out, which leads to a smaller 'gene pool' as well as a much greater sense of community. I am going to consider three of these communities that are now quite widely discussed on-line. There are other groups that have been included by others, but three populations have quite well-documented information.

Okinawa, an archipelago about 580 kms off the coast of Japan boasts the top number of *proven* centenarians. The proportion is about 0.6% of the total population of 1.3 million people. These elderly Okinawans are also much healthier than other very old people and they mostly remain vigorous and healthy despite their extraordinarily advanced years.

Sardinia, where the second population live, is a large, rugged island that is about 193 kilometers off the western coast of Italy and here, the men who are mostly shepherds are especially long-lived. In one town of 1700 people, five, that is 0.29% of the population are more than 100 years old.

Like the Okinawans, these Sardinian men are very active because of their need to walk through their rugged landscape but they are also relaxed and drink small amounts of red wine throughout the day.

Ikaria is another Mediterranean island that is part of Greece but 36 miles off the coast of Turkey. This population also has a very high rate of centenarians and good health. Ikaria has well-known mineral hot springs, the health effects of which will be discussed in a later chapter. Again, we see a population of people who are active throughout their lives, especially through walking, farming and fishing. They have low rates of chronic diseases, low rates of cancer and cardiovascular disease and exceptionally low rates of dementia.

Diet in long-lived populations

There has been considerable effort to identify the optimal diet for healthy aging and there is no doubt that every researcher brings some of their own bias to the study. It is rarely possible to be accurate about what people ate fifty, seventy or even more years ago, when many of the key elements of their current health occurred. The data for the Okinawans is probably the most accurate and most extensively studied and here it is compared with the Japanese diet of the same era. The biggest differences are highlighted.

There do not seem to be equivalent studies conducted for the long-lived Sardinians and the only data I could find was an example of a daily meal plan for healthy centenarians. This included breakfast of milk and bread; lunch of pasta and vegetables; dinner of eggs, chicken, legumes and vegetables plus wine, olives, olive oil and water.

In a study of Ikarian men and women aged 80 or more[23], there is more detailed data that is summarized in the table. As far as diet is concerned, it is be difficult to find many consistencies between the groups other than that they all have a reasonable intake of oils. In the two Mediterranean groups this is olive oil, and in the Okinawans, sesame oil. Both these oils are rich in oleic acid.

[23] Panagiotakos, Desosthenes B et al (2011) Sociodemographic and lifestyle statistics of oldest old people (>80 years) living in Ikaria Island: The Ikaria Study. Cardiol. Res. & Pract. Doi:10.4061/2011/679187

The other two stand out but very different 'foods' are the local sweet potatoes in Okinawa that make up a huge proportion of their food and coffee in Ikaria! The Okinawa purple 'sweet' potato is apparently extraordinarily rich in anthocyanins, even higher than blueberries and they are the staple food here. Coffee on the other hand is also rich in antioxidants, especially a polyphenol called chlorogenic acid and is reported in some studies to reduce the risk of Type 2 diabetes, Parkinson's and Alzheimer's diseases. The Okinawan people also have very low rates of hormone-dependent cancers, including breast, ovarian, prostate and colon cancer whereas the Japanese, as a nation, have only lowered rates of ovarian and prostate cancers. We don't know the rates of these cancers in the Ikarians and Sardinians but both Greece and Italy have relatively high rates of breast and prostate cancers.

These three countries are healthy by world standards but there is still much to learn as the next chapters will show.

FOOD	Okinawa, 1949	Japan, 1950
Grains - rice	154 (12)	328 (54)
Grains - wheat etc.	38 (7)	153 (24)
Nuts & seeds	<1 (<1)	<1 (<1)
Oils	3 (2)	3 (1)
Legumes	71 (6)	55 (3)
Fish	15 (1)	62 (4)
Meat (incl. poultry)	3 (<1)	11 (<1)
Eggs	1 (<1)	7 (<1)
Dairy	<1 (<1)	8 (<1)
Sweet potatoes	849 (69)	66 (3)
Other potatoes	2 (<1)	47 (2)
Other vegetables	114 (3)	188 (1)
Fruit	<1 (<1)	44 (1)
Seaweed	1 (<1)	3 (<1)
Pickled vegetables	0 (0)	42 (<1)
Alcohol & flavors	7 (<1)	31 (2)

Factor – Daily diet of those aged 80 & older	Ikarian Men	Ikarian Women
Energy intake (kcal/day)	1425 ± 532	1087 ± 460
Alcohol (mL/day)	186 ± 181	117 ± 114
Coffee (mL/day)	339 ± 260	293 ± 228
Tea (mL/day)	109 ± 84	97 ± 90
Food times/week		
Olive Oil	6.8 ± 2.7	5.3 ± 2.5
Cereals	1.7± 2.5	0.9 ± 1.7
Fruits	5.5 ± 3.1	3.9 ± 2.7
Vegetables/salads	4.8 ± 2.8	3.5 ± 2.8
Legumes	2.0 ± 1.5	1.3 ± 1.1
Fish	2.1 ± 1.6	1.5 ± 1.2
Potatoes	3.3 ± 0.9	3.1 ± 0.8
Sweets	1.2 ± 2.4	1.3 ± 2.1
Red meat & products	1.8 ± 1.9	1.2 ± 1.4

Chapter nine

CROSS CHECKING RESEARCH RESULTS

So much information and collective wisdom and risks of bias!

I doubt that most people realize how much of what we hear about science and medicine is selective. This doesn't necessarily mean that it is biased or incorrect but just that there is a huge amount of work being undertaken and the results that reach the public are only a minute proportion of the whole. Furthermore, we never hear all the details of any study because for reasons of practicality everything is summarized and as we know from experience of life 'the devil is in the detail'.

Most research today is conducted by teams of investigators who usually receive funds from some type of research granting body. If you are not a well-known researcher or you work alone, it is generally difficult to obtain funding in science/health. Moreover, it is nearly impossible to receive funds to research a new or different idea unless you have already obtained some results to prove your concept. These limitations were initially introduced to try to ensure that research funds were allocated to worthwhile projects and worthy investigators, but they can risk the types of disastrous outcomes that I will describe in the next chapter.

Most of the research conducted by individual research teams is published in journals. There are currently 5,235 journals that are published by '*Index Medicus*'. These journals are not all about health by any means, but a high proportion are. Most research journals publish about once a month and each monthly publication contains about 15 academic papers. In most cases these papers have been reviewed by at least two 'peer' reviewers who are *supposedly* both unbiased and experts in the research area.

In the last few years 'open access' publishing has become more common and this form of publication makes the research available for everyone to read at no cost to the reader, but generally at quite high (financial) cost to the researcher. Open access publication has some obvious advantages to researchers, but it can result in at least two unfortunate outcomes. The first is that research groups who have more money and can afford to pay, have their research read at the expense of those who can't afford to pay. The second is that some very poor-quality research has been published by journals who primarily exist to make money. Nevertheless, even conventional publications of large international studies can lead to biased interpretation and devastatingly bad results.

Despite our best efforts, since there is no possibility of anyone assessing all the literature in any area, there are real risks that some poor research will gain favor and some valuable observations and theories will be overlooked. There are also many examples – like the cholesterol story below – where very good researchers make bad mistakes and the voices of the critics aren't heard until it's too late; sometimes they aren't heard at all!

Use of the 'Grey Literature'

In addition to the peer-reviewed, published literature, there is also the so-called 'grey literature', which consists mainly of reports issues by governments and both private and public organizations.

There are many international bodies such as the World Bank, The United Nations and the World Health Organization who work together and with governments, universities and research organizations to not only provide an extraordinary service to all of us, especially to developing countries, but who also write many valuable reports and provide access to international data. There is little doubt that the information contained in the grey literature is as accurate and unbiased as possible but not all the conclusions drawn in the reports is unbiased as the people writing the reports are quite likely to be influenced by the 'opinions of the day'.

The Tables of foods shown in the last chapter are examples of data from the 'grey literature' and in the next section I will also use data from various international bodies to examine some of the assumptions about health. As I've already suggested, these records can sometimes reveal discrepancies that lead us to question assumptions that might have been made when researchers start a project with an outcome in mind.

Chapter ten

'WHERE ANGELS FEAR TO TREAD?'

Cholesterol studies & the fate of the much-maligned egg

Most published scientific and medical findings are highly tested and valid. Yet, it is not unknown for one incorrect concept to become popular and for other, important and correct work to be rejected or overlooked.

As I suggested in the last chapter, if an idea is unusual or takes a different angle from the popular view, it might take a great deal of time before the alternative idea is even considered or the idea might become permanently buried. Furthermore, when an idea from science is translated through to public policy, *massaging* of the initial idea by governments and various bodies with vested interests can do a great deal of harm.

One example of over-massaging the original idea is seen in the 'Seven countries study' led by an American physiologist *Ancel Keys (who died aged 100 in 2004)*. Keys set out to find the cause of cardiovascular diseases (strokes and heart attacks in particular) and he observed that the people of the Mediterranean region not only had a high rate of centenarians but low rates of cardiovascular illnesses. This led Keys to establish the first ever multinational epidemiological study in 1958, whose results showed that *blood serum cholesterol* levels correlated with heart attacks in *six* of the *eight* countries. It also appeared to show (from five to 40 years of follow-up work) that there was a correlation between total serum cholesterol and coronary heart disease and that that was associated with an increased risk of death from cancer. The scope of the work was very impressive so it is depressing that such a great deal of work by so many researchers could have been incorrectly interpreted!

The observations that the studies made on the association between total blood cholesterol and cardiovascular disease was (possibly) 'sound' – why didn't anyone ask why the association was NOT found in two of the eight countries i.e. 25%? - but even more importantly, the extrapolation that raised blood cholesterol was caused by the intake of dietary cholesterol seems to have been yet another unfounded assumption. Sadly, the dietary advice that emerged from this study has had some devastating consequences on the world's health!

Interestingly, the study results on fats seemed to be supported by the early US Framingham Heart Studies and this led to advice to people not to eat eggs. As a result, eating eggs became controversial from the late 1960's and people in the 70's (in the USA) were even trying to develop low cholesterol eggs.

Keys and his research team had no evidence to support their assumption that *dietary cholesterol* was the cause of raised *blood cholesterol*, but he and his colleagues convinced the powerful American Heart Association that eating fat was the cause of the problem. The Heart Association then convinced a USA Government Committee to recommend that the American population adopt new dietary guidelines and in 1977, the Committee produced guidelines: 'Dietary Goals for the USA' that advised:

(a) reducing fat, saturated fat and cholesterol consumption and (b) increasing carbohydrate consumption to 55-60% of the diet.

Other western countries, including Australia, adopted these new guidelines and I can readily recall that in the 1970's we all adopted a diet that included a great deal of rice, pasta and bread. Most of us also soon noticed that we were putting on a great deal of weight! Interestingly – and I don't know what influenced this – but plate sizes and serving sizes also increased in Australia from the early 1980's onwards.

I have used a document produced by the United States Department of Commerce called 'Food Consumption, Prices and Expenditures 1970-1993' to produce four diagrams that show how the consumption of protein (meat, chicken and fish), eggs, animal fat versus vegetable oils and flour & cereal products, changed as a result of the 1977 guidelines. The decline in egg consumption began earlier as a result of worldwide publicity.

The advice might have been 'incorrect, but people certainly followed it!

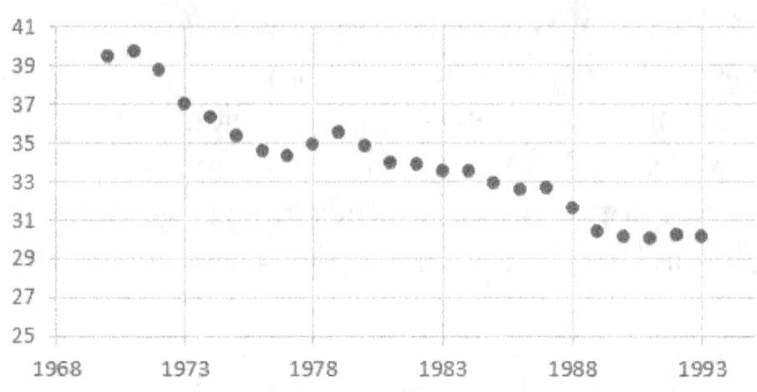

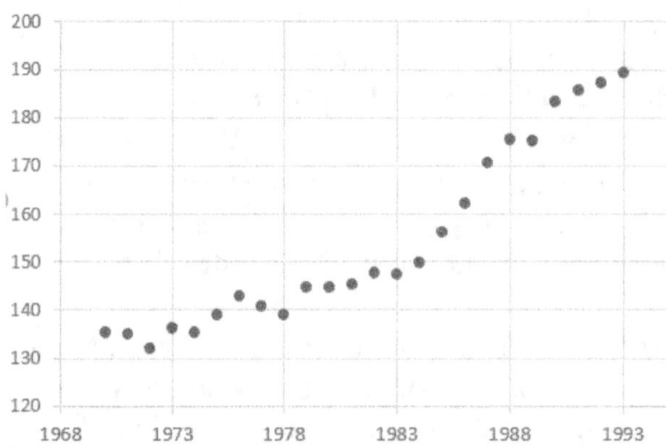

Unlike the egg consumption that was affected earlier, the advice to increase carbohydrates started with the 1977 guidelines and it is easy to see the massive change that occurred. A food pyramid that showed the proportions of carbohydrates that 'should' be consumed made it easy for people to adopt the new diet.

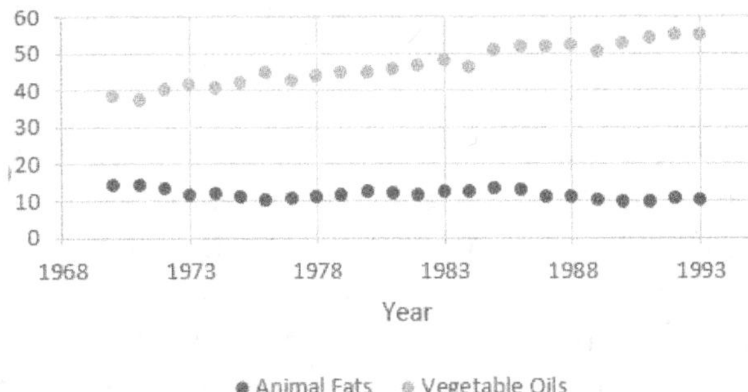

People were also advised to eat margarine instead of butter and to cook with vegetable oils. Sadly, the importance of Extra Virgin Olive Oil was completely 'lost in translation'! This resource doesn't identify the types of vegetable oils but Canola (originally developed from Rapeseed) became a major new agricultural product in the early 1980's. Since 1995, most of the world's Canola crops are genetically modified so consumers might have a slightly higher intake of the herbicide glyphosate when eating Canola Oil. However, probably the most undesirable aspect of Canola Oil is that doesn't contain the desirable oleic acid.

There was also no emphasis on eating fish (or fish oil) in this research so fish consumption didn't change but people were discouraged from eating too much red meat and it is easy to see that poultry replaced red meat whilst the total intake of protein stayed constant.

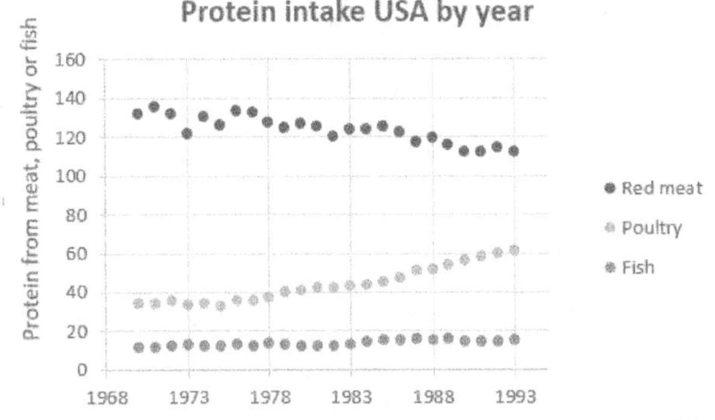

Milk and cheese

Somehow the messages about fat consumption were lost when it came to dairy foods or possibly consumers were tricked by advertising. But whereas consumers switched to drinking low fat (dairy) milk, many replaced this milk fat by consuming more cream products and as a result milk fat intake increased from 5.6 lbs. per person per year in 1980 to 8 pounds per person in 1993.

Eating Italian food was widely promoted, but this was interpreted through *fast food* marketers and 'sold' to the US market as pizza! So, consumption of cheese more than doubled from 11.4 pounds per person in 1970 to a high 26.3 pounds in 1993.

It turns out that eating dairy food might have advantages for some populations as we will see when we look at the world statistics on individual diseases. However, the *specific* dairy products that we consume are probably of great importance.

Fruits and Vegetables

The message to eat more fruits and vegetables resulted in slight increases in each group and the total change was an increase from 566 pounds in 1970 to 675 pounds in 1993.

Problems with extrapolation of data and resultant poor health outcomes

Although there was a reduction in cardiovascular deaths in the US from the 1970s onwards, this could largely be accounted for by three other factors:

(1) The introduction of the '*statin*' drugs to control cholesterol

(2) The genetic identification of the familial hypercholesterolemia gene and the management of individuals at high risk

(3) The improvement of emergency procedures in ambulances and in hospitals.

It has also been proven that smoking adversely affects levels of the 'good' high density lipoprotein HDL – so there are more factors than diet contributing to cholesterol, but smoking will be discussed more in a later chapter.

Eggs

The egg producers suffered globally from the misinterpretation of the earlier research but since there is now a great deal of evidence to show that eggs are a highly nutritious food and that the cholesterol consumed in food does not raise blood levels of cholesterol, egg consumption is on the rise again.

In the meantime, the adoption of diets that are high in sugar has greatly raised the rates of, and deaths from diabetes. Diabetes is also increased by the widespread use of air-conditioning but more about this later! From 1985 to 1989, the rate of diabetes in 65-year old persons was 0.7% but between 1990 and 1999 it rose to 1.06% and from 2000 to 2011 it rose further to 1.6%.

The overall result of the over-zealous and incorrect interpretation of the early research results on diet has been huge as it has not only led to extremely bad and expensive outcomes (in terms of health), but it has denigrated research in the eyes of many consumers. Furthermore, in retrospect it is easy to see that the conclusions about dietary fat should never have been drawn since in at least two of the countries in the original studies, Denmark and Norway where the incidence of heart disease is low, diets are rich in fat. Conversely, in Chile the diet is low in fat, yet the incidence of heart disease is high! Nevertheless, this discrepancy doesn't mean we should rush out and eat diets that are high in fat.

Chapter eleven

WORLD DEATHS FROM CANCER & 'CHRONIC' ILLNESS: THEORIES VERSUS DATA?

How world statistics differ from the messages we are given

At the end of the first chapter, I mentioned that whilst the Okinawan people have (or at least had) very low rates of the three most frequent hormone-dependent cancers, breast, ovarian, prostate as well as a low rate of colon cancer, the Japanese as a nation, have only lowered rates of ovarian and prostate cancers. This is probably a lifestyle factor, but it could also be genetic. There is no way we can tell conclusively from the information I have considered thus far.

The rates of these three cancers are not available for either the Ikarian or the Sardinian people but both Greece and Italy have high rates of breast and prostate cancers. In the next Table I show the rates of these cancers in a few example countries to highlight the differences between countries and between different types of cancer in each country. Please note that these data are from 1996 and that life expectancy has risen considerably since 1996 in most countries. However, my reason for including this Table is to highlight both the differences between countries and the differences between different diseases in the same country.

Clearly one lifestyle might protect against one disease but not necessarily another.

Location	Age/Life Expectancy	Breast Cancer	Cancer Ovary	Cancer Prostate	Cancer Colon
Okinawa	81.2	6	3	4	8
Japan	79.9	11	3	8	16
Hong Kong	79.1	11	3	4	11
Sweden	79.0	34	10	52	19
Italy	78.3	37	4	23	17
Greece	78.1	29	3	20	13
USA	76.8	33	7	28	19

The Table above shows the Hormone-dependent Cancer and Colon
Cancer Deaths per 100,00 people that is obtained from each of Data
from the World Health Organization, 1996 and the Japan Ministry of
Health & Welfare, 1996

*Note: In the original publication, colon cancer was listed as a hormone-
dependent cancer but there is only weak evidence that this is the case. I
have used three tones to differentiate the low (white), medium (light
grey) and high (dark grey) rates of these cancers in the seven
areas/countries. All these countries are regarded as having low rates of
Ovarian Cancer.*

When we are presented with results like these, we immediately observe
the differences and most researchers have tended to assume that the
differences are caused by one or more of 'genes', 'dietary intake', 'other
aspects of lifestyle such as exercise, alcohol drinking and/or smoking'.
However, research often ignores, or is unable to measure many sub-
categories of these factors – such as types of alcohol, methods of
cooking, methods of heating houses – and is also unable to measure or
disinterested in assessing a great many other environmental factors that
might be contributing to the cancer risks.

So, whilst it is moderately well established that genes, diet and 'lifestyle'
are strong contributors to many health conditions, we need to realize
that research is limited either by the available existing data – often
information that has been collected in national records and/or by what
is *easily measurable.*

Information that is easily collected is often very limiting because there
are more aspects of life and the variability of day to day living that can't
be measured than those that can be measured. Moreover, unless data is
collected in a laboratory, researchers depend on people's memory and
honesty; neither of which is reliable.

When looking for environmental factors such as chemical exposures, researchers usually rely on finding 'clusters' of affected people. This can be exceptionally difficult because people who share the same environment don't necessarily receive the same exposures. Furthermore, and probably more importantly, since at least some of the factors that induce cancer are likely to occur many years, often decades before the cancer is diagnosed, a person's current life and lifestyle, and even location might not be relevant to their illness.

Because of all these many limitations on human based research, much of the useful research on cancer has been undertaken in laboratory animals where despite the many obvious limitations, the results are reliable within the context of the experiments. The animal results are especially helpful when testing for genetic factors as many human genes can be mimicked by animal genes. However, since humans invariably lead much more complex and varied lives than caged animals, there are huge numbers of variables that cannot be tested.

So, thinking beyond the well documented and important lifestyle factors of diet, exercise and tobacco use, we shouldn't overlook home heating and cooling, 'air fresheners' and cleaning agents and radiation of various types, not to forget possible exposures to chemicals and metals through air, water and soil. Even 'light pollution' (excess light at night) is now emerging as a possible cause of several illnesses. Then as well as excesses, we might also consider possible mineral deficiencies that might cause illnesses.

Factors related to 'climate' and 'migration' are important – for example a dark-skinned person living in a region with low light levels will suffer from Vitamin D deficiency while a fair skinned person moving to the tropics is likely to develop skin cancer. These are obvious adaptations but there may be many more subtle differences that no-one has yet considered.

We also should consider the types of homes that people live in and how much exposure there might be to constant light and air-conditioning? It is well known that shift-workers are more susceptible to many illnesses but how much difference does it make if there is quite bright ambient light at night when you are genetically adapted to living in a cave?

Sleep and stress are both now known to be important factors in all health problems so how can we compare the stressed life of a person living in the middle of a busy city with someone living a simple, traditional life on an idyllic island? Nevertheless, the Hong Kong people were doing well in 1996!

Identifying key predisposing factors for the highest world death rates

I have included data taken from 182 countries and a Table of Diseases from **worldlifeexpectancy.com** both to emphasize the diversity of factors that affect health and to identify some changes that we can make to improve our own health. Many of the key factors are currently ignored or trivialized, and some are unknown, but this brief analysis of the figures suggests that some important factors are currently being ignored – often for political reasons. There are also several examples where very negative aspects of lifestyle protect people from some of the diseases associated with 'affluence'.

Data from the World Health Organization from 2016 shows that Coronary Heart Disease and Stroke are the highest causes of death and account for 15.2 million of the world's 56.9 million deaths per year. Diabetes accounts for 1.6 million deaths and Dementias more than doubled between the years 2000 and 2016 such that dementia is now the 5th highest cause of death compared to the 14th highest in the year 2000.

Since this book is about aging, I have focused on age-associated diseases and so have ignored the infectious diseases and AIDS that aren't specifically associated with aging. I also haven't included pulmonary diseases as I think it is well established that they are associated with smoking and air pollution of various sorts. I am assuming that everyone who is interested in health knows about these and tries to avoid them!

The Table of Diseases on the next page has been taken from World Figures of 182 countries published by **worldlifeexpectancy.com**. Numbers represent the world ranking for deaths from each of the diseases and not incidence as above. Each line shows the countries with the highest and second highest incidences and then the rates for Japan, Spain and Australia. But again white – high numbers are (relatively) 'good' and dark grey – 'low numbers' are the worst. This is a competition you don't want to win. In the text that follows I will reveal the countries with the lowest rates of each illness and explain why I think that this is so.

Disease	Rank 1	Rank 2	Japan	Spain	Australia
Coronary HD	**Turkmenistan**	**Ukraine**	182	175	173
Stroke	**Indonesia**	**Sierra Leone**	157	175	177
Diabetes	**Fiji**	**Mauritius**	180	159	152
Parkinson's	**Finland**	**Ireland**	42	25	15
Pancreatic Cancer	**Kazakhstan**	**Uruquay**	6	43	47
Alzheimer's	**Finland**	**Kuwait**	158	29	28
Colon Cancer	**Hungary**	**Slovakia**	32	21	44
Breast Cancer	**Tonga**	**Grenada**	149	115	93
Prostate Cancer	**Saint Vincent**	**Antigua**	149	113	83

I found these results very interesting and often surprising. I wondered what they are telling us they we haven't already been told and what we could learn from them if we thought about the *outstanding* and/or *unusual* features of each of the countries with the **highest** rates of each disease and compared this with the country with the **lowest** rates.

Coronary Heart Disease

Highest rates: Turkmenistan, Ukraine
Lowest rate: South Korea

Characteristics of the countries with highest and lowest rates

Turkmenistan is quite a physically large country in South-Central Asia that is mostly occupied by the Karakum Desert. Only about five million people live here and although it is formally denied, the country has cholera, AIDS and the plague. Turkmenistan was part of the Soviet Union until 1995 when the Soviet Union broke up.

The Turkmenistan diet is rich in dumplings and pies that are cooked in cottonseed oil, which although it is relatively high in saturated fat has recently been shown to reduce cholesterol. Turkmenistan is known for its melons, which are supposed to be good for the heart as is their standard drink of green tea. Vodka is the alcoholic drink of choice.

Possibly the worst health factors In Turkmenistan are polluted drinking water and extremely high levels of industrial and agricultural pollution.

Ukraine is also previously part of the Soviet Union, the Ukraine is in Eastern Europe, west of Russia. Typical foods include the famous borshch and like, Turkmenistan, dumplings. There are a great variety of alcoholic and non-alcoholic drinks in the Ukraine, especially high-quality wine. A study conducted by the World Bank (2010) sought to explain the high death rate in the Ukraine. They reported that every third Ukrainian aged 18–65 had a high blood pressure, about 29% of the respondents were overweight, and approximately 20% were obese.

Like Turkmenistan, and in both cases a legacy of the previous regime, the Ukraine has *exceptionally severe air pollution* in the industrial cities and there is *chemical pollution* from agriculture in soil and water throughout the country.

So, are the world's highest death rates from cardiovascular disease more likely to be due to pollution or diet-related obesity caused by an excess intake of dumplings and alcohol? In fact, both diet and pollution are probably contributing factors but given that the Ukraine is only 40/51 and Turkmenistan 50/51 in the rankings for obesity in the European region (WHO, 2008), it seems as if pollution may be a key risk factor in both countries?

In support of this, a recent study has identified air pollution as a major cause of cardiovascular disease[24]. Obesity is likely to be a compounding factor, but it seems probable that the highly toxic physical environments push these two countries to the top of the world list.

But given that industrial pollution (sadly) is a growing factor in many countries, perhaps a more helpful question is which country has the lowest rate of cardiovascular deaths? Furthermore, can we use this information to reduce our own risk of cardiovascular disease?

[24] Rajagopalan S et al (2018) Air pollution and cardiovascular disease. J. Am. Coll. Cardiology. DOI:10:1016: J.JACC.2018.07.099

It turns out that one answer to lowering cardiovascular disease risk could be relatively simple, but it is not something that I've personally ever heard spoken about.

South Korea is the country with the lowest rate of deaths by cardiovascular disease and this is <u>despite</u> South Korea having quite high rates of air pollution. The answer seems to lie in their intake of **Kimchi**, which is eaten with every meal. Kimchi is a fermented blend of cabbage, chilli, scallions and other spices and as well as having high levels of Vitamin A and C and lactobacilli, it has particularly high levels of Vitamin K2. Japan, which has the second lowest rate of cardiovascular disease has a similar food, called Natto.

Vitamin K2

If you haven't heard of Vitamin K2, you are not alone. Although this form of Vitamin K was suspected to exist, it has been researched quite thoroughly in the last few years, but you may not find K2 on the shelves of most shops that sell vitamins.

I will expand on Vitamin K2 in a later section but for now you should know that it is well established in the *recent* scientific literature that both *vitamin D* and *vitamin K2* are essential for cardiovascular health – as well as for preventing osteoporosis. These vitamins ensure that our calcium is integrated into our bones rather than remaining in our arteries where it will cause cardiovascular disease!

A large study undertaken in the Netherlands, called The Rotterdam study investigated the occurrence and causes of diseases in the elderly. The studies of heart disease showed that anyone who consumed more than 200 micrograms of vitamin K2 each day had up to 57% less risk of dying from cardiovascular disease than those who consumed less. Other studies have shown that the risk of death from CVS drops by 9% for every 10 micrograms of K2 intake per day.

What is quite complicated about the K2 research is that there are different forms of the vitamin and that those with longer chemical chains (Mk-7, Mk-8 and Mk-9) last longer in the body. Kimchi has a short chain K2 and needs to be eaten at least once a day, so for most of us, other sources of K2 are likely to be more readily available.

Japanese Natto is the best source of K2 but it is an 'acquired taste' and is only eaten in some parts of Japan. In 'Western countries, cheese is probably the highest source of K2 and especially the longer chains. BUT not all cheeses contain Vitamin K2 and you will find a Table of Vitamin K2 rich cheeses in a later chapter. It seems that low K2 intake may be yet another poor outcome of the 'low fat' research discussed above. It is apparent that many full cream dairy products are excellent sources of K2.

Stroke

Highest rates: Indonesia, Sierra Leone
Lowest rate: Canada

<u>Characteristics of the countries with highest and lowest rates</u>

Stroke is a condition where blood supply to the brain is disrupted. Sometimes it is accompanied by bleeding but not always. Infections are commonly detected after stroke, but the medical literature is somewhat divided on whether infections might cause stroke?

If we consider the two countries in the world with the highest rates of stroke, Indonesia and Sierra Leone, we see that they are both tropical countries with frequent flooding and many areas of swamps. As is typical of such tropical countries they have animals like monkeys, chimpanzee, hippopotami, crocodiles and tsetse flies and malarial bearing mosquitoes.

Both Indonesia and Sierra Leone have extremely high rates of infectious diseases including malaria, dengue fever, hepatitis A (to name just a few) and very high rates of bacterial contamination in water. Since the link with infection and stroke has already been made, it seems likely that, at least in these countries that the major causes of strokes are likely to be infectious agents. It is also probable that many different types of infections cause strokes.

But now to look at why Canada has the lowest international incidence of death by stroke? In fact, Canada's own resources describe stroke as one of their leading causes of death but at 18.2 it is a great deal lower than Indonesia's 186.29/100,000 deaths.

The food that stands out as being almost an emblem of Canada is **Maple Syrup** and this is a classical ingredient of a Canadian breakfast. It is high in sucrose (67%) but it also has high levels of *Riboflavin* (vitamin B2) and *Manganese*. Indeed 100 gm of maple syrup has slightly more than the recommended daily intake of each of these nutrients.

Each of these nutrients is likely to play a role in reducing strokes: Riboflavin plays a key role in lipid metabolism and deficiency in riboflavin compromises our important detoxifying enzyme *Glutathione-S-Transferase*. But while riboflavin has many important roles in brain function and aging, the enzyme *manganese-dependent superoxide dismutase* plays a special protective role in vascular function and people with chronic stroke have a genetic change that reduces the function of this enzyme.

This is not to suggest that you should rush out and take more manganese as it is a trace element and adults only requires about 2 mgs each day, but it is very important to have a good daily intake of all B vitamins as because they are water soluble, they are not stored in our bodies. However, as long as you buy *authentic* Maple Syrup and only have a little, it is a very pleasant and inexpensive way to top up on essential nutrients!

Diabetes

Highest rates: Fiji, Mauritius
Lowest incidence in Belarus

<u>Characteristics of the countries with highest and lowest rates</u>

Fiji and Mauritius are both island countries in the South Pacific and
Indian oceans respectively. Both are unpolluted, beautiful lands with
tropical climates that are around 20 – 22 C in the dry winter months
and just a little hotter but more humid in summer.

Fiji's population is about 900,000 while Mauritius is slightly larger at
1.265 million people. Both populations are known for their happy
disposition and tourism is a major industry in both places. They each
have sugar as a major industry, so the availability of sugar is probably
high. The indigenous cuisines in both countries are quite diverse but
despite this, increases in 'fast food' over the last few decades have
played havoc with the health of these populations and obesity is
prevalent.

Obesity is associated with diabetes II, yet it is not generally regarded as a
direct or 'sufficient' cause. Furthermore, although Fiji has the 23rd
highest world rate of obesity, in Mauritius, obesity is relatively low,
although rising, at 10.8%.

So, what other environmental factor is common to these countries that
might interact to cause diabetes?

Well, what is immediately striking about the two countries is the lack of
variation in ambient temperature throughout the year. It is never cold!
Is it possible that these idyllic conditions might increase the risk of
diabetes? It seems they might!

Supportive evidence comes from data that shows that rate of diabetes has increased in countries throughout the world soon after air-conditioning is introduced. That is, with air-conditioning, people who live in cold countries no longer need to experience cold! It was initially thought that the association between air-conditioning and diabetes might be attributable to lowered levels of Vitamin D, because people then spent more time indoors. However, there are extensive studies in rodents and now some in humans[25] that show that *exposure to cold* is necessary to activate brown adipose tissues. Furthermore, it is well established that this *metabolically active brown fat tissue* is important in the prevention of diabetes.

The world's lowest death rate from diabetes is found in Belarus, which is not by most standards, one of the world's healthiest places to live. Belarus suffered badly from the fall-out of the 1986 Chernobyl accident and that nation's coal burning has generated air pollution that is one of the highest in the world. Childhood mortality due to Carbon Monoxide from indoor stoves is very high and the rates of alcohol and tobacco use are one of the highest in the world. But – possibly because homes have only been heated by relatively inefficient stoves in winter, diabetes is not prevalent.

So, whilst living in a constant temperature in 'paradise' is extremely pleasant, it is probably not as good for preventing Diabetes as having to adapt to some variations in temperature, especially to cold. I am not suggesting for a moment that diet isn't also important in preventing diabetes as we know that diabetes has risen in association with the intake of 'junk food'. Nevertheless, for most of us a bit of shivering should help increase our brown fat and reduce our risk of diabetes.

---

[25] Saito M et al (2009) High incidence of metabolically active brown adipose tissue in healthy adult humans: Effects of cold exposure and adiposity. (In Diabetes Publish Ahead of Print, published online, April 28, 2009

Parkinson's Disease

Highest incidences Finland, Ireland, USA, high incidences in Australia and Spain.
Lowest incidence is in Moldova

<u>Characteristics of the countries with highest and lowest rates</u>

Although there may be some individual susceptibility and other chemicals may also be involved, there is considerable evidence from the top research institutions linking Parkinson's disease to agricultural chemical exposures. In California (US) *paraquat, maneb* and *ziram* have all been linked to Parkinson's disease not only in farm workers but in people who lived close by and *Benomyl,* which was banned in the US ten or so years ago is still linked to cases there because of its persistence in the environment.

I approached the question of possible exposures in Finland and Ireland by looking at the top crops in the two countries and their most frequent pests. Both Rye in Finland and Potato in Ireland are beset by *Fusarium root rot* and this (at least until recently) has been treated with *Benomyl. Benomyl* was banned for use in Australia in 2006 but like in America the chemical probably remains in the environment. The chemical also seems to be readily available for purchase on the Internet, so it is obviously still in use in some countries.

Benomyl works by linking to microtubules. These are the tubules that pull chromosomes apart during cell division, but which also play a key role in the transmission of signals in nerves.

Benomyl has been linked to birth defects, and it is not at all surprising that it would also be linked to Parkinson's Disease.

Moldova, a small landlocked European country that was once part of the USSR, has the lowest incidence of Parkinson's Disease. Moldova used to be known as the 'Garden of the Soviet Union'; 75% of the country is fertile and the soil is well-endowed with minerals. Currently 21% of the farms are owned by individuals and 61% by co-operatives, and there is low use of fertilizers and pesticides, which used to be supplied by the Soviet Union.

Pancreatic Cancer

Highest incidences in Kazakhstan and Uruquay
Lowest incidence in the Maldives

<u>Characteristics of the countries with highest and lowest rates</u>

Kazakhstan in central Asia is the world's largest landlocked country and was also a previous Soviet State. The country has low population density – about 18.3 million people in total – and is rich in oil, gas and minerals. Kazakhstan also breeds sheep, horses, cattle and camels and preserves most of the livestock products by <u>curing and smoking the meat.</u>

In contrast, Uruquay is a Spanish speaking country that has the reputation of being the most peaceful country in South America. Like Kazakhstan, Uruquay also breeds cattle and sheep and it exports combed wool, rice, soybeans, frozen beef, malt and milk. The diet includes high quantities of <u>cured and smoked meats</u> as well as delicacies like *chimchurri* sauce that amongst other ingredients is rich in garlic and parsley.

Unfortunately, a high intake of red, especially processed red meat has long been suspected as a key factor in pancreatic cancer and these world incidence statistics strongly support this. The risk of pancreatic cancer increases about 1.2 times with every increase of 50 gm per day consumption of processed meat.

The Maldives, which has the world's lowest death rate from pancreatic cancer, eats a diet that is primarily based on coconut, fish and starches such as rice, taro, sweet potato and cassava. Much of their fish is cooked before eating but some tuna is cured through a process of boiling, smoking and drying in the sun.

The difference in the risk for pancreatic cancer is likely to be due to the balance of high-quality starches in the diet and the intake of fish rather than meat, especially cured meat!

Alzheimer's Disease

Highest in Finland and Kuwait
Lowest in Singapore

<u>Characteristics of the countries with highest and lowest rates</u>

Unlike the other diseases I have considered above, it is much more difficult to understand the variation in Alzheimer's disease by country. There are certainly genetic factors involved in susceptibility but the countries with the highest number of cases also show some strong geographical patterns. I wondered whether these patterns might reflect gene dispersion by migration in past centuries or whether the factors are more related to climate and/or local environmental factors?

Australia and New Zealand form one high incidence group, the Middle East and Northern Africa form a second, the countries on the western side of Europe (Spain, France, UK, Scandinavia) form a third group of geographically linked countries – which are only separated by water from the second group, and then Northern America including USA and Canada form a third group.

El Salvador, Peru and Myanmar are the only geographically disconnected countries that have a very high incidence.

All the North African countries (Morocco, Algeria, Tunisia, Libya and Egypt) are in the highest incidence group whereas, in the Middle Eastern countries Turkey, Syria and Lebanon all have a very high incidence. Since the incidence is much lower in both Cyprus and Israel, I wondered whether these countries might reveal any secrets?

A recent detailed genetic study of the population of Cyprus shows that although they are genetically diverse, the people have shared ancestry with the people of southern Italy. If we were to judge the genetic theory based on this fact alone then it wouldn't be supported because Italy has a much higher incidence of Alzheimer's (23.13 deaths per 100,000) compared with Cyprus (14.97 per 100,000). But culturally Cyprus seems to be divided between the Greek and Turkish speaking peoples and again their rate of Alzheimer's is not a match with either: Greece is 31.36, Turkey is 51.11.

There may be many different factors involved in the development of Alzheimer's and some researchers have suggested that early life exposure to *lead* might be a major cause? On a similar theme of heavy metals - many recent studies have found high levels of *inorganic copper* in the *blood* of Alzheimer's patients and these researchers propose that this is likely to have come from drinking water. They also point out that the wide introduction of copper pipes throughout the world might account for the rise in Alzheimer's disease and its curious association with highly developed and wealthy economies.

Other researchers have proposed that it is lead rather than copper that is the problem and that individuals who are exposed to lead in childhood and this is born out in humans and in aged (23-year old) monkeys who were exposed to lead as infants. But the evidence suggests that both lead and copper can affect brain development and function, and other heavy metals including mercury and cadmium have also been implicated.

Alzheimer's and plumbing?

Some of these heavy metals are found in polluted air but lead and copper may often be transferred through water pipes and thus imbibed. Finland, who have the highest incidence of Alzheimer's have special problems with their plumbing because of the extreme weather conditions. An article on the internet from the *Helsinki Times* called 'pipe renovations are at hand' showed some typically damaged pipes and stated that 'pipe leakage led to the greatest proportion of reimbursable household damage in Finland. They estimated that in this decade there would be an average of 10,000-15,000 pipe renovations per year.

This led me to wonder why Russia, another country with similar weather, has quite a low incidence of Alzheimer's disease and the 'sad reason' is probably that a large proportion of Russian homes don't have any indoor plumbing!

Singapore has by far the lowest rate of Alzheimer's in the world at only 0.4. In 2016, the Singapore National Water Agency PUB was interviewed about the possibility of there being heavy metals in their water supply. Their response was impressive and other countries might like to take a similarly responsible approach. Here are their key points:

- They conduct more than 400,000 water quality tests each year
- All rooftop water tanks are tested at least once each year

- The water supply is a network of corrosion resistant pipes such as cement-lined ductile iron pipes and copper pipes
- There is systematic replacement of all pipes regardless of the age of the housing development!
- Lead soldering is banned
- ALL plumbing pipes and fittings must comply with all the regulations before they can be advertised, displayed or offered for sale.

Singapore is sometimes criticized for the rigidity of its regulations, but it seems that this responsible attention to detail could be the reason for their vastly reduced rate of Alzheimer's disease if Alzheimer's is indeed associated with copper leaching from pipes?

Ovarian Cancer

Highest rates in Kazakhstan (13.62) and Brunei (12.95)
versus the lowest Mozambique (0.87)

<u>Characteristics of the countries with highest and lowest rates</u>

This is the second cancer where Kazakhstan has the highest incidence
in the world and the other was Pancreatic cancer. There is apparently a
genetic link between the two diseases, even though the pancreas and
ovary seem to be unrelated organs? The genes, BRCA1 and BRCA2
GIVE INCREASED RISKS OF BREAST, OVARIAN AND
PROSTATE CANCERS AS WELL AS OF PANCREATIC
CANCER.

BUT DESPITE ANY GENETIC RISK FACTORS, LIKE
PANCREATIC CANCER, OVARIAN CANCER RISK IS ALSO
INCREASED BY CONSUMING CURED MEATS. SO, IT SEEMS
LIKELY THAT BOTH EXTREMELY HIGH CANCER RISKS IN
KAZAKHSTAN ARE CAUSED BY THIS CUSTOM.

The reason for the high risk in Brunei may also be related to a relatively
high dietary intake of one or more cured foods. Brunei people have a
high dietary intake of fish but because their fish supplies are
inconsistent, they have quite a high intake of smoked and cured fish. In
addition, one of their staples is a fermented shrimp paste called
Belacan. One detailed resource showed that Brunei *Belacan* is often
insufficiently dried to prevent the growth of molds and yeast and so it
could be such contaminants rather than the fermentation process that
underlies the cancer risk?

So, if in contrast to looking at the countries with the highest incidence of ovarian cancer, we look at the country with the lowest levels of this cancer we find Mozambique. Mozambique is rich in precious metals but a country living in poverty. 97% of their agriculture is undertaken by individual (mostly) women-headed families using hand cultivation. They are known to use traditional varieties of crops, especially the disease-resistant Cassava and 80% of their diet is composed cereals and the starchy root Cassava. Malnutrition and vitamin deficiencies are frequent in this impoverished country but not surprisingly Ovarian Cancer rates are low.

Colon Cancer

Highest in Hungary and Slovakia and
lowest (again) in Mozambique

<u>Characteristics of the countries with highest and lowest rates</u>

Both Hungary and Slovakia have similar diets that have a high proportion of dairy, cheese and meat together with both salty and sweet baked goods comprising many different types of 'highly prized' buns and pastries. Hungarian Goulash is a well-known, tasty meat dish that is heavily flavored with paprika and Hungarian (winter) salami and smoked pork are also staples.

Traditionally, Hungarians eat a large breakfast that is an 'open sandwich' filled with fresh butter, cheeses, cream cheese and/or preserved, cured meats. They also eat some vegetables, sauerkraut, soured peppers and gherkins.

I think that we've all been warned enough about low fiber diets as risk factors for colon cancer to not recognize this traditional diet as being highly risky! By comparison, poverty-stricken Mozambique with its subsistence diet of high fiber, locally hand-grown crops, has a very low risk of this disease as do most of Africa and South Asia!

Breast Cancer

Highest in Tonga and Grenada
Lowest in Bhutan

<u>Characteristics of the countries with highest and lowest rates</u>

Tonga is a Polynesian paradise – an archipelago of 169 islands of which only 36 are inhabited. Two thirds of Tonga's agriculture comprise the root crops *Taro, Sweet Potato* and *Cassava* but they also grow bananas and coconuts. Together with neighboring Nauru, they have the highest rates of obesity in the world.

Grenada is another island country that grows bananas but is in the West Indies. Here, the people are mostly of African descent and like the people of Tonga, they are becoming obese. In most if not all countries of the world where bananas (in particular) have been grown, the soils are heavily contaminated with pesticides. Furthermore, pesticide residues also affect the development of obesity, so the association of obesity and breast cancer is not fortuitous. Organochlorine pesticides have recently been shown to be accumulated in breast cancer tissue[26] but whether carcinogens ever remain in bananas is unclear? Much of the literature suggests that the flesh of bananas is safe to eat but everyone is encouraged to eat only organic bananas in order to reduce the risks to the environment and farm workers.

[26] He TT, Zuo AJ, Wang JG, Zhao P (2017) Organochlorine pesticides accumulation and breast cancer: A hospital-based case-control study. Tumour Biology doi: 10.1177/1010428317699114.

In contrast to the highly contaminated regions of banana plantations, Butan has the lowest rates of both breast and prostate cancer. Butan has a plan to become totally organic but does currently use some pesticides. Interestingly there is a report on the internet from July 2016, where Butan regulators banned the import of chilies that were contaminated with organochlorine residues so it appears that Butan is ahead of most countries in its diligence about organochlorine contamination and this would certainly be in keeping with its world's lowest rate of breast cancer.

Prostate Cancer

Highest Saint Vincent and Antigua,
like breast cancer, the lowest rate is in Bhutan

<u>Characteristics of the countries with highest and lowest rates</u>

The medical literature does not show clear links between organochloride exposure and prostate cancer, but most studies on prostate cancer have been restricted to blood samples and negative studies on blood plasma are very likely to be irrelevant. Organic compounds are known to accumulate in fat so samples of adipose (fat) tissues, where chemicals accumulate over time, or prostate tissue itself need to be used to investigate this.

If we just consider that the world's highest incidence rates are in two islands in the West Indies region, where banana plantations use high levels of organochlorines and that near-by island communities have the highest incidence of breast cancer, it is very likely that organochlorines are also involved with prostate cancer. Moreover, since the lowest rate is in Bhutan, it is difficult not to conclude that the same causative factor is involved.

As further support to the high risk of prostate cancer in regions where banana plantations prevail, three Australian postcodes (2452, 4860 and 4883) show raised deaths rates due to Prostate Cancer of 1.23x, 1.47x and 1.35x respectively.

The next Table summarizes the conclusions I have drawn from the world data but <u>please note</u>:

Most if not all the diseases listed are almost certainly multifactorial – that is, they have several different, often compounding causes, several of which may not be listed here. Furthermore, it is well known that an extremely large number of genes alter an individual's susceptibility to any disease and that stress can probably exacerbate any other risk factor.

Nevertheless, the use of these world figures gives an insight to the real causes of several of these diseases and these causes are not commonly discussed.

Apart from the conclusions I have drawn by looking at the figures and thinking about their meaning, there is rigorous, published research findings that supports all the information presented here.

Disease	Probable primary Cause	Possible factor(s) that lowers risk
Coronary HD	Air pollution	Vitamin K2
Stroke	Infectious diseases	Mn, B2 (riboflavin)
Diabetes	Lack of sufficient exposure to cold + excess dietary sugar	Low sugar diet & (some) exposure to cold
Parkinson's	Chemical exposure especially Benomyl	Low exposure to herbicides – especially Benomyl
Pancreatic Cancer	High intake of cured/smoked meat	Diet that is low in cured/smoked meat
Alzheimer's	Exposure to metallic copper & lead through plumbing	Government regulations & upgrading of plumbing infrastructure
Ovarian Cancer	High intake cured/smoked meat plus? herbicides	Low use of herbicides, Low calorie, high fiber diet
Colon Cancer	High fat, low fiber diet	Low calorie, high fiber diet
Breast Cancer	Organochlorines (banana plantations)	Organic 'philosophy'
Prostate Cancer	Organochlorines (banana plantations)	Organic 'philosophy'

PART C

LIFESTYLE - ACTIONS WE CAN TAKE TO REDUCE AGING AND AGE-RELATED OUTCOMES

Chapter twelve

LIFESTYLE, LIFE EVENTS AND TELOMERE LENGTH

Chromosomes:
What we currently know about telomere length

Most people will have heard of DNA, genes and chromosomes and that they are important in the traits that we inherit from our parents. Strangely enough, although each of the many thousands of genes is individually important, the ends of the chromosomes that are called TELOMERES, and that DON'T convey any specific genetic information, play a critical role in determining length of life.

Telomeres are the special regions found at each end of each chromosome, somewhat like a boundary fence. They are comprised of the sequence of six DNA bases – TTAGGG (thymine, thymine, adenine, guanine, guanine and guanine) -but telomeres don't function as single sequences and are referred to in thousands of bases or kb's.

Studies that have been undertaken of the length of babies' telomeres at birth find that the length is quite variable between individuals and ranges between about 10,000 and 20,000 base pairs (bp) per 'chromosome end'. In theory, the baby with telomeres of an average length of 20,000 bp will have a much longer life expectancy because regardless of the starting length, the number of base pairs per telomere reduces to about 4,000 bp towards the end of life.

From this information alone, it's easy to see that some individuals appear to start off life with approximately twice the life expectancy of others. However, because of the impossibility of the task of analyzing the telomere length of a human population for an entire lifespan, no studies have proven that this relationship between telomere length at birth and lifespan is true in humans. Nevertheless, all the data collected thus far is consistent with this being the case and in all animals with much shorter lifespans where telomere length has been studied, this relationship between initial length and lifespan has been proven.

So, not only does telomere length at birth predict our lifespan but on average telomere length declines more rapidly in men than women. This increased rate of reduction in males occurs over the lifespan and the more rapid loss may be due to hormonal effects.

Based on observations on telomere shortening, women should live longer than men and population data has always shown that this is so. In the past, most researchers have thought that the difference was due to lifestyle differences but recent data from the UK has shown that whilst the gap between men and women has narrowed, falling from 4.2 years in 2006-8 to 3.7 years in 2012-14, it hasn't changed since then.

In the UK, average life expectancy for women at birth is now given as 82.9 years, and for men it is 79.2 years. Nevertheless, this discussion is about *averages* and there are certainly many men with longer than average and many women with shorter than average telomeres.

Telomere length at birth

Studies from several different tissues taken at birth show conclusively that an individual starts off with a 'personal telomere length' that is constant between the different cells of their body. Moreover, there are no apparent differences in telomere length between males and females at birth.

An individual's personal telomere length is probably influenced by hundreds of genetic factors, but one known effect is paternal age. For every extra year of a father's age, a child's telomeres increase by 22 bp so if you happen to have 'chosen' an older father, you will have started off with somewhat longer telomeres and might expect to live longer. Sperm telomeres lengthen with paternal age and so the egg is fertilized by sperm with longer telomeres. However, while an older father may give the child some telomeric advantage, dominant gene mutations (some with very negative effects) also increase in older sperm so overall, increasing paternal age is probably not an advantage to offspring.

Many laboratories have studied the length of telomeres in men and women and the results of one study from France are reproduced in the Figures shown in this chapter. These data were obtained from white blood cells using a DNA technique that measured the length of the telomeres.

The statistical analysis from this French study shows that the females in this study have slightly longer telomeres than males (8.67 kilobases versus 8.37 kilobases) and although telomeres were reduced by aging in both males and females, the yearly rate of attrition was also slightly less in females than males (0.036 kb per year versus 0.038 kb per year).

If you were to draw a 'trend-line' through the middle of the points on these data, you would find that the average matches the lengths given above and that the female data looks slightly higher than the male, but a notable feature of the data is the 'scatter'. There are no males over 70 who have telomeres that are longer than those of the males under 30 but there is one young female with a telomere length that is more typical of the women aged 50-70, and shorter than half of those aged over 70.

The consensus of all the research that has been conducted indicates that both genetic and lifestyle factors contribute to telomere length.

Some implications of reduced telomere length

Further proof of the critical role of telomeres in defining lifespan has come from experiments with mice. Mice that are genetically deficient in telomere length have shortened life spans and interestingly, they also have increased rates of cancers.

Mice with short telomeres are less able to heal wounds or to recover from damage to their bone marrows. The specific changes that occur prior to death due to telomere shortening are the characteristics of extreme old age.

These characteristics of extreme old age are:

- Breakdown of the walls of the small intestine
- Reduced ability of white blood cells to divide and hence reduced immunity
- Wasting away of the spleen
- Abnormal blood picture

Telomere length and age-related diseases in humans

There is a vast literature about measurements of telomere length and its association with age-related health problems in humans. I will list some of the larger studies without attempting to provide any of the thousands of references. All studies take age and gender into consideration and all give consistent results. Shortened telomeres are found in these conditions:

- Insulin resistance and hypertension (Framingham Heart Study, USA)
- Diabetes and stroke (Cardiovascular Health Study, USA)
- Systematic reviews of the medical literature show that there is an inverse relationship between telomere length and the risk of coronary heart disease. This risk includes specific events such as myocardial infarction, stroke and the progression of atherosclerosis. Individuals with telomere length in the shortest of four quartiles had 1.54 times the risk of cardiovascular disease as those in the highest quartile of telomere length.
- Cancer, especially bladder (sub-groups), digestive system, lung, urogenital (NIH funded studies, USA)

How important is telomere stability?

Although telomere length is the basis of aging, sometimes length *per se* isn't <u>always</u> the most important factor in telomere function. It is a fact that short telomeres are usually associated with less stability than longer telomeres but since some long telomeres can be unstable, some researchers suggest that might *also* be important to be concerned with telomere stability. For example, patients with Alzheimer's disease don't invariably have shorter telomeres, but their telomeres have significant signs of dysfunction and at least in this disease, dysfunction might be more important than the length?

Recent studies from lower organisms and plants show that special (RNA) molecules are involved in the stabilization of telomeres and similar systems are probably also involved in human cells. So just having long telomeres is certainly not all that is needed for good cellular function.

Telomerase activity is retained in some adult cells

Telomerase is a cellular enzyme that increases the length of telomeres, **but this doesn't mean that taking telomerase will make you live longer!** Although most of the earliest publications on telomeres and telomerase only detected the enzyme telomerase's activity in <u>cancer cells</u> or equivalent, several more recent studies have detected telomerase activity in some (apparently) normal cells in blood. Telomerase activity is also found in some of the cells of some rapidly renewing tissues. However, in these special cells, the level of enzyme activity is usually less than that found in cancer cells and its activity is probably very tightly controlled.

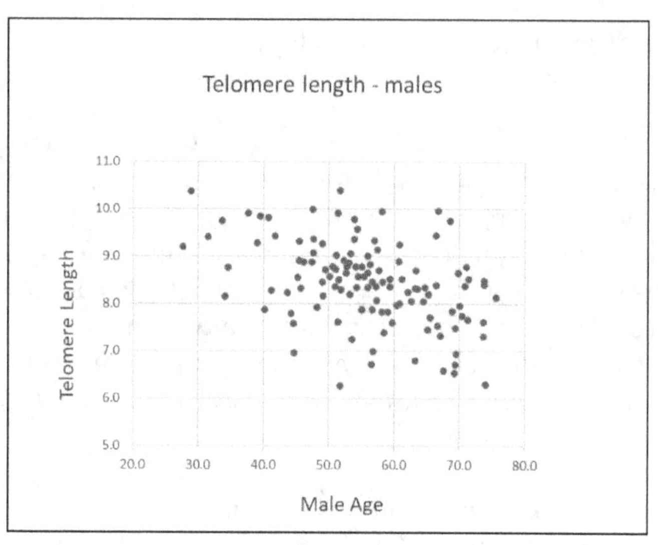

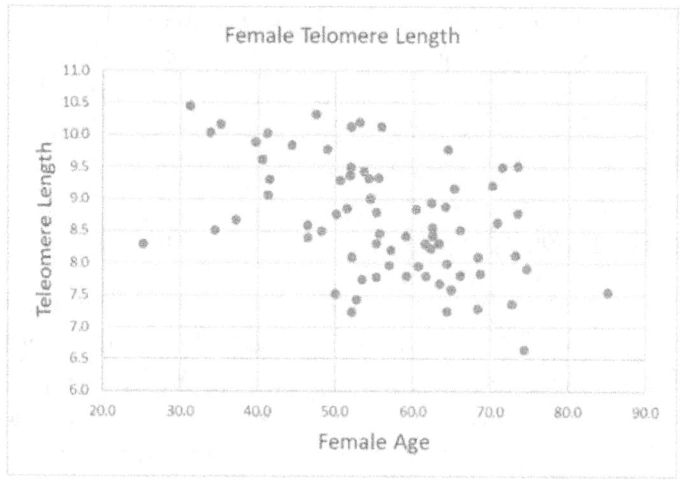

Telomere length by male and female age – data is reproduced from Benetos A et al (2000): Telomere length as an indicator of biological aging[27].

---

[27] Reproduced from *Hypertension http://www.hypertensionaha.org*.

Why telomeres shorten under normal conditions

Because of the way DNA is replicated, using one strand as the template while having a lead RNA primer attaching ahead of the polymerizing process, there needs to be a 'buffer zone' ahead of the replication and the telomere unit provides this disposable buffer. The loss of telomere length *per cell division* should be about 20 bp but actual rates are between 20 and 100 bp and the reason for this isn't completely clear. However, if we work with this figure and take an average of (say) 50 bp loss per cell division then each cell could have the capacity to divide between 120 and 800 times depending on how many bases an individual started with.

In most cells, the telomeres just diminish with cell division over time until they reach the telomere limit, when the p53 gene is activated and the cell becomes senescent or apoptosis system is activated and the cell self-destructs. I am not going to talk about these mechanisms here BUT it is important to understand that *whenever* cells become senescent, they cause INFLAMMATION, and this accelerates the aging process.

Infections and telomere shortening

Since telomere length is such an important marker of our potential lifespan, we need to understand how we can best protect it.

I have scanned some of the very large numbers of studies that have measured telomere length and some of the helpful findings are:

Early life infection has a pronounced effect on telomere length. A study from the Philippines *prospectively* collected early life data on infections in 1,759 individuals and then tested their telomere length when they were young adults aged between 21 and 22 years old. They found that telomere length was most affected by 'more than average number of infections (especially diarrhea) experienced between six and twelve months old. Infant diarrheal infections predicted a 45 bp loss in telomere length, which was the equivalent of about 3.3 years of adult telomeric aging in their population[28]. In this study, 'more than average' was rated as one standard deviation above the average rate.

A study of the effect of persistent infections of cytomegalovirus (CMV), herpes simplex virus type 1, herpesvirus type 6 and Epstein-Barr virus (EB) was undertaken in 400 otherwise healthy adults (aged 53 to 76 years) over three years. The EB virus showed no association with telomere length but each of the other viruses showed *very large effects*, each shortening telomeres by the equivalent of more than three years. Being CMV seropositive was associated with the equivalent of about 12 years attrition. These associations were not affected by age, sex, employment type, body mass index or smoking!

---

[28] Eisenberg DTA et al (2017) American J. Human Biology **https://doi.org/10.1002/ajhb.22962**

Environmental toxins and telomere length

Several environmental and occupational exposures are associated with telomere shortening. These include:

- Traffic-related air pollution (i.e. particulate matter, black carbon, benzene and toluene)
- polycyclic aromatic hydrocarbons (PAHs),
- N-nitrosamines,
- Pesticides
- Lead
- Various mixed chemical exposures in industry
- Hazardous waste exposure

Longer telomeres are not always good

Exposure to arsenic and persistent organic pollutants (POPs) are associated with longer telomeres but not in a 'good' way. Rather it is accepted by most researchers that arsenic interferes with the telomere in a way that is carcinogenic.

Apart from the finding that arsenic and POP exposures lengthen telomeres, there may be some genetic associations between longer telomeres and cancer risk? In a report from the Female Asian Lung Cancer Consortium, the group found that a specific genetic variant in the TERT gene that is associated with longer telomeres gave a 50% increased risk of lung cancer in never-smokers.

The TERT gene is the gene that elongates telomeres in the reproductive and embryonic cells. This gene is usually switched off in most other normal cells apart from having a role in repairing some chromosomal repair. However, TERT is usually switched **ON** in cancers and plays an important role in carcinogenesis.

Epigenetics and telomeres

I am deliberately going to omit any detailed discussion of a whole relatively new field of genetics 'epigenetics' that might eventually lead to key developments in aging research. The term epigenetics literally means 'outside genetics' and it is mostly a study relating to the proteins that bind to DNA to form the chromatin of chromosomes. Many of the changes that occur in this attached protein are passed through generations and so are inherited but not in quite the same way as genes.

There is no doubt that the epigenetic modifications of genes are essential to normal development and that they are susceptible to environmental influences, some of which may be involved in cancer. However, although epigenetic modifications may influence the rates of telomere attrition, there is no doubt that telomeres are the final determinants of aging and lifespan.

Chapter thirteen

ACTIONS TO AVOID AGE-RELATED DISEASES

What can we do to avoid age-related diseases?

Several studies on lifestyle and telomere length have demonstrated that specific lifestyle factors are associated with telomere shortening so eliminating/changing these deleterious factors should reduce the shortening although this is not necessarily the case. A huge Danish study[29] that measured telomere length, ten years apart in over 4,500 people found that short telomere length was associated with (a) increased age, (b) current smoking, (c) increased body mass index and (d) physical inactivity.

Some other habits for telomere length preservation that should also be considered relate to general care of our organs and tissues. I am going to list a few here but this list is not exhaustive and not all these areas have been studied with respect to longevity per se. Nevertheless, the only ways our cells can deal with infection and repair involves cell division and cell division gradually reduces the length of telomeres. So, we should try to reduce wastage by eliminating or reducing unnecessary cell division.

[29] Weischer M et al (2014) Telomere Shortening Unrelated to Smoking, Body Weight, Physical Activity, and Alcohol Intake: 4,576 General Population Individuals with Repeat Measurements 10 Years Apart PLoS Genet 10(3): e1004191

Daily habits and telomere length

Make sure you never get burnt and try to avoid too much sun exposure.
This is an obvious way of protecting the health of skin. Whenever we
allow ourselves to get burnt by the sun, we stimulate the underlying skin
cells to grow. For this reason, people with white skin who live in hot
environments often have such aged skin. As a person of European
background who has lived in Australia for most of my life and
participated keenly in outdoor sports for most of my life, I have much
older-looking skin than (say) a person of similar heritage living in
England or a darker skinned person living here. I have been playing golf
for about 10 years and only wear a glove on my left hand. Consequently,
my right hand looks much older than my left hand.

Despite my continuous sun exposure, I am in the one third of people of
my age who has not (yet) had a skin cancer. I wondered whether this
might be because I have been taking one cod liver oil tablet daily for the
last forty years. There are many claims for cod liver oil offering some
protection and I suspect it is because of the high level of vitamin A.
Vitamin A protects the health of all epithelial cells – i.e. the cells of all
your 'outside' and 'inside' linings.

Try to *protect yourself from any unnecessary cuts and wounds*. Some
ways of doing this are making sure that you wear appropriate protection
when undertaking any activities that expose you to risk.

Potentially risky undertakings might include everyday activities like walking through bushland as much as gardening or undertaking 'handyman' activities of any type. Protection during gardening and handyman activities are especially important because you are likely to be exposed to toxic substances as well as risking cuts and abrasions. But, remember that every scratch will use up precious and irreplaceable cell divisions.

Avoid infections!

This may seem like an obvious thing to do but it is amazing how many people just accept that catching the latest virus is inevitable when if you are careful it should not be. Here are some suggestions of how to reduce your chances of avoiding contagious illnesses:

Avoid crowded places

Public transport is probably not the best option at times when illnesses are prevalent so ideally you will avoid it. But when you can't, these suggestions might help.

First MAKE SURE THAT THE INSIDE OF YOUR NOSE IS WELL-LUBRICATED. Noses become very dry in overheated environments and especially in airplanes. If you keep the inside of your nose lubricated with products made for this, or even Vaseline, you will find that have considerable protection against infection.

Wearing a facemask might look as if you yourself are infected but it is a very effective way of reducing your chances of being infected by the flu and other respiratory infections. Studies in hospitals have shown that if the staff wear face masks, their rate of infection from patients is very low.

Keep yourself very well hydrated

Ideally carry some type of filter if the only water you can access isn't good quality but don't ever let yourself become dehydrated. When you are well hydrated, your immune cells can move through your blood more rapidly as your blood viscosity is lower. Cells must have *adequate hydration* and *balanced pH* to function normally.

It is easy to observe how plants wilt in hot weather and either fail to grow or become 'sick' if the soil hasn't the correct nutrients or hydration, but plant cells are more resilient than our own cells partly because they have a cell wall. So, you can imagine how insufficient nutrients and dehydration might affect us.

Wash your hands regularly and thoroughly! Also, dry your hands thoroughly after washing them.

Wet hands pick up and spread contamination much more readily than dry hands. If washing your hands might be difficult, carry some cleansing wipes. Cleansing wipes are also good to clean the various dubious surfaces that you might have to touch throughout your any journeys. I'm not suggesting being paranoid about this, but wipes will help you stay well when you are required to travel in places where infection is prevalent.

If you are dining out, *select food which is very unlikely to be contaminated.* In some countries this means avoiding fish, which might not have been refrigerated adequately at some stage. In other places this will mean only choosing fruits that are served with the skins on so that when you remove the skin yourself, you can be reasonably sure that the inside is uncontaminated. You are also usually safer choosing food that you can see being freshly cooked and most importantly, the food that everyone else is eating. Eating the local food is usually a safe option, especially if the venue is very popular.

I would like to be able to assume that your food hygiene at home is exemplary but if your family suffers from occasional gastrointestinal infections then you should look carefully at what you could be doing wrong? Keeping food too long or at incorrect temperatures is a common source of problems but re-use of the same surface for uncooked and cooked food (especially chicken) is probably the most common food hygiene error.

The temperature and air quality of your home and/or other regularly visited places can also be a large contributor to ill health. There are three main reasons for the health issues: (i) People regularly overheat buildings in winter and often overcool them in summer and these extremes of indoor temperature are undesirable. (ii) There is often insufficient turnover of air, oxygen levels are reduced, and carbon dioxide and other exhaled gases are too high. (iii) Many people remain in their outdoor clothes when they move into an indoor environment that requires quite different attire. These are easy things to correct but are common causes of minor illness.

How you manage your home environment will be very individual, but I would encourage you to use ceiling fans rather than air conditioning wherever it is feasible for cooling. Similarly, fans can be used to circulate the air in rooms in winter to distribute the heat from various types of heat sources. This will almost always allow you to reduce the heat that needs to be generated at the heat source and will reduce energy costs as well as eliminating temperature extremes in various parts of the heated space.

It is also important to remember to retain adequate humidity indoors. Whilst too high humidity can cause mold and other problems, too low humidity can dry out cellular membranes. If your room is becoming dry, especially if you are heating with gas, you will find that just having a vase or reasonable size vessel of water will be helpful.

As mentioned in the earlier section, most environmental pollutants are associated with significant telomere shortening.

A recent study gives an exact estimate for exposure to cadmium: for each 1 µg/L serum cadmium, leucocyte telomere length is decreased by 3.74 bp. One Occupational Health & Safety reference states that the recommended reference range for workers in their study was $\leq$ 5.0 µg/L.

Cigarette smoking seems to be a major source of blood cadmium so apart from all the other negatives you already know about smoking, you should not only NOT smoke yourself, but you should avoid being exposed to others' smoke.

The risks associated with smoking were known in the late 1800's so if you still smoke, you are a very slow learner. You need to work out why you smoke? If it's an oral fixation, then chew some gum because chewing stimulates your brain. But do give up because smoking negatively effects all parts of your body and you really smell bad as well!

Use indoor plants in your home to remove pollutants, especially if you use gas or wood burning stoves. NASA has studied the air-cleansing properties of many indoor plants and although most remove some pollutants, the *Peace Lilly* is a very good all-rounder that is difficult to kill!

Alcohol and telomere length

Increased alcohol intake did not affect telomere length in the Danish study, but alcohol dependence was associated with an almost 50% telomere length reduction in a Japanese study. The latter study also found that the reduction was worse if there was a vitamin B1 (thiamine) deficiency.

These results seem to be quite different, but they probably don't reflect differences in research techniques but rather, they are a cautionary tale about GENES AND ETHNICITY.

There are large racially based differences in the ability to metabolize alcohol that are conferred by the *alcohol dehydrogenase* genes. Racial genetic differences mean that in 90% of Oriental people, liver levels of the nuclear *alcohol dehydrogenase* gene are much higher than in Caucasians whereas 50% of Oriental people lack the second ALDH2 gene, which is a mitochondrial gene. This means that Japanese people metabolize alcohol differently to Caucasians and so the results of the two studies cannot be compared.

Ideally no one should drink alcohol to the point of intoxication but even for moderate drinkers, this is a reminder to make sure that if your drink that you have an adequate intake of vitamin B1 (in particular). If you find that you are easily intoxicated by alcohol, it is a sign that you shouldn't drink it at all.

Stress

Both short periods of acute stress and sustained chronic stress have been found to shorten telomeres. Stress itself is associated with high levels of inflammation and this may be the cause of the telomere length reduction.

I will write more in a later chapter about strategies for minimizing stress. But perhaps the most important message about avoiding infections is to avoid stress.

Whenever we are stressed, either from extreme exertion, or from an upsetting emotional experience (or worry), our immune systems are suppressed. We are then very vulnerable to any 'threatening' virus or other infectious agents. So, if you are stressed, make sure you stay away from infectious people!

It is difficult to study nutrition in populations of people and some of the data on nutrition measures blood or tissue levels of nutrients rather than food intake. This is often a reasonable estimate but can sometimes mask another factor. To date, the following conclusions have been drawn:

- Deficiencies in Magnesium and vitamin D have both been proven to be associated with short telomeres.
- Low intake of Omega 3 fatty acids was associated with greater telomere shortening over five years.
- Consumption of processed meat was also associated with telomere shortening.
- Higher plasma levels of folate were associated with longer telomeres.
- Vitamin D, multivitamin use and higher intake of foods containing vitamin C and E were all associated with longer telomeres.

In summary

The good news is that most of the advice we've been given about being healthy is supported by studies on telomere length. We should eat well, take vitamins whenever our food doesn't supply adequate amounts of vitamins and minerals to meet our daily needs, undertake plenty of exercise, not smoke, never drink to excess and not become stressed and our average telomere length should be appropriate for our age.

Our health can be even better if we apply more of the lessons from the world population-based findings that I've discussed above but there is still more to consider!

Chapter fourteen

STARTING AT THE HEAD

ORAL AND DENTAL HEALTH - OUR MOUTHS - A RESERVOIR OF INFECTION!

Oral and dental health

We know that having recurrent infections reduces the telomere length and hence the longevity of our immune cells, but many people don't realize that their teeth can easily undermine their other efforts to be healthy.

'The teeth are the only non-shedding surfaces in the body, and bacterial levels can reach more than 10^{11} (i.e. 100 billion) microorganisms per mg of dental plaque'[30]

---

[30] Li, X et al (2000) Systemic diseases caused by oral infection.

This quote and the remarkable figures are from a research publication entitled 'Systemic disease caused by oral infection' that is referenced below. I am sure that you, like me, are absolutely astounded by the vast numbers of bacteria that could be there, waiting to launch themselves into my bloodstream should my gums become inflamed.

Rates of tooth decay vary between countries and races but as an estimate, in the USA the rate of periodontitis is 47% in 30-year old's and 70% in 65-year old's! Infections originating in the gums could be causing or at least exacerbating many other illnesses and so our dental health needs to receive our regular attention.

The bacteria in the mouth don't usually enter into the bloodstream unless the gum tissue becomes broken but bacteria are frequently released after a dental procedure and this is why, if you are having surgery that will involve a prosthesis (such as a hip replacement) the surgeon will/ or should test you for existing infections beforehand and eliminate any that are there before the surgery. You should then make sure that you don't visit the dentist before the operation and subsequently take care with any future dental work.

What are the risks of infection following dental procedures?
The combined results from 11 studies show the following rather worrying results. Bacteremia (the presence of live bacteria in the circulating blood) was observed in:

- 100% of people after a dental extraction – (other than 'third-molar' i.e. wisdom tooth removal to prevent crowding)
- 70% after dental scaling
- 55% after third-molar, wisdom tooth, surgery removed to prevent crowding (i.e. no evidence of infection beforehand)
- 20% after endodontic treatment

Clinical Microbiology Reviews 13: 547-558

Another study of 735 children undergoing dental treatment for extensive tooth decay found that nine per cent of them had detectable bacteremia (infection in the bloodstream) prior to the dental treatment.

Root canal procedures

There are some articles on the Internet such as one from a society of endodontists that claim that it is a myth that root canals cause illness. I am going to quote part of one such statement: '*This false claim was based on long-debunked and poorly designed research conducted nearly a century ago, long before modern medicine understood the causes of many diseases.*' The same article claims that saving your natural teeth, if possible, is always the best option.

Whilst I hope that most people who have a root canal procedure do not suffer, the statement above is clearly incorrect. This is easily seen from the results in the published review that I have quoted as well as from the data in many other very recently published, scientific papers.

In contrast to the 'endodontists society', the article on *Colgate.com* is responsible and balanced. This points out that 'root canal complications' are a risk and that bacteria can remain in a root that hasn't been treated or that there might be a small crack in the root of the tooth that is easily missed and can lead to bacterial growth.

The root canal procedure is performed, after all, to remove diseased tooth pulp and to fill and seal off the area, and whenever we are dealing with infectious tissue there is a risk that the infections will spread.

To date there are limitations in the current endodontic disinfection protocols, and advanced disinfection techniques designed to reduce the microorganisms and biofilms in chronic infection are still being improved.

It is well established that both dental procedures and oral infection itself can cause an infection of the heart valves called bacterial endocarditis. This is a rare disease in people with normal hearts but people with some pre-existing heart defects are at risk if bacterial infection occurs. Unfortunately, the connection between the oral cavity and endocarditis was originally missed because sometimes the oral infections occur months or even years before the endocarditis is obvious.

It is universally accepted now that dental procedures can be the cause of endocarditis, but whilst their role in many other illnesses is highly likely, and supported by substantial international research, the studies on some diseases don't yet meet all the rigid criteria and so are not yet quite accepted as proven.

In the following conditions oral infection is *extremely* likely to be a causal factor for *some* but not all affected people:

- Coronary heart disease
- Atherosclerosis
- Myocardial infarction
- Stroke
- Bacterial pneumonia

Oral infection is also frequently involved in pregnancies that result in low birth weight and since dental health is compromised by the raised hormones in pregnancy, attention to dental health during pregnancy is important.

As we grow older our gums recede because the number of cells that can divide is reduced. So, whilst excellent oral hygiene is important at all ages, it is imperative as we age. Daily tooth flossing or some other type of interdental cleaning is advisable as well as very thorough tooth cleaning two or more times each day. For people who are unable to floss, mouth washes can achieve the same types of bacterial removals, but long-term use of mouth washes might have some negative effects and mechanical techniques are probably safer.

Many well-controlled studies have been undertaken to test which types of toothbrushes clean best and although all toothbrushes are somewhat effective, there is overwhelming evidence that oscillating and/or rotating electric-powered toothbrushes are far superior to 'manual' brushes. There seem to be some small differences between the manual brushes of different design but not enough to be concerned about which one you choose as your 'back-up' or travelling toothbrush.

Daily flossing and twice a day thorough cleaning (or more if you like) will help retain the health of your gums and thus reduce the need for the gum cells to divide and this in turn will help you stay not only healthy, but alive!

Some of the benefits of dental and gum health have to do with retaining the cell numbers in your gums and thus their capacity to divide but because healthy gums stop mouth bacteria from entering our blood, they also reduce the load on our immune cells. Keeping the rate of infections as low as possible restricts wasted cell turnover in our immune system.

Evidence that there is a massive benefit of having healthy gums as you age comes from many studies such as the following one conducted in California. In this study (results published in 2011) the investigators examined the relationship between dental health and death (by any cause) in 5611 older Californian adults, over a period of about nine years. Those who never brushed their teeth at night had a 20 – 35% increased risk of death compared to those who brushed every day. Never flossing increased the risk of death by 30% compared with flossing every day. Not visiting a dentist at least every 12 months increased the risk of death by 30-50% and mortality was also higher in people who had less than 20 teeth!

A note about vitamins and dental health

I will discuss vitamins and whole-body health in a later chapter, so I'd just like to point out here that nutrition and specific vitamin intake is critical to your oral health. I am just adding a note here to inform you that vitamin K2 together with enough vitamins A and D can *not only* inhibit but apparently can reverse dental decay. However, at this stage we don't know how long it takes, how much you need to have nor how bad your decay can be at the start.

The importance of keeping and using your teeth

Apart from avoiding the pain of tooth ache and avoiding the often, lethal infections that originate in the mouth, retaining and using your teeth has other huge benefits. These are driven by the acts of biting and chewing, which are of course the purpose of teeth.

Chewing, saliva: taste and digestion of food

During chewing the salivary glands secrete saliva that is mostly water but also very importantly electrolytes and enzymes amylase (that digests carbohydrates) and lipase (that digests fats). There are also some other cells and antimicrobial chemicals that we won't consider here but saliva also acts as a solvent for substances that confer taste so without it, foods not only can't be digested properly but they also don't have appropriate taste.

The act of chewing produces more saliva and as well as promoting the first phases of digestion, the chewing breaks the food into smaller amounts and the saliva initiates swallowing.

Hyposalivation (reduced production of saliva) is a side effect of some medications and this can put elderly people at great risk. They can have greatly reduced ability to masticate and swallow their food as well as not receiving the benefits that saliva plays in reducing oral infections.

Food manufacturing practices and unforeseen outcomes

Apparently, all chewing is not equal! A study that involved subjects chewing three types of bread that the authors described as 'industrial', 'artisian' and 'wholemeal', tested how much saliva and salivary maltose were present in food boluses after a standard period of chewing. There were considerable differences between subjects but there were also significant differences in the rate of uptake from the different breads. Industrial bread was greatest then artisian and then wholemeal.

To me, these results suggest that eating so-called industrial bread is likely to lead to a person absorbing more calories than from the other types of bread. This might be undesirable for younger people but quite desirable for the elderly who could (usually) benefit from receiving more calories per chew!

Traditional Sourdough versus Industrial Bread

This comment is not restricted to aging but whilst researching bread and chewing, I discovered that all types of <u>industrially</u> produced bread use the 'baker's yeast' *Saccharamyces cerevisiae,* which results in bread with high levels of gluten. In contrast traditional sourdough bread uses one of the *Lactobacilli* in its processing and does not generate a reaction in gluten-intolerant people, even when the dough has some wheat content.

It seems likely that the rise in gluten intolerance is caused not only by the increase use of wheat in bread-making flour but also by the current industrial processes.

Chewing and brain stimulation

Another important, slightly indirect but critical finding about aging and health is that the act of chewing has a very important effect on the brain. When we chew, we activate many different regions of the brain so just receiving nutrition – through (say) liquid meals – will result in reduced brain function. There is far more to chewing than just the nutrition that usually results.

This is a relatively new field of research, but the findings are very encouraging. It has been established[31] that loss of the ability to chew, acts as a source of chronic stress and by activating the hypothalamic-pituitary-adrenal (HPA axis) induces:

- Cognitive impairment
- Cardiovascular disorders
- Osteoporosis

---

[31] Azuma K et al (2017) Association between mastication, the Hippocampus and the HPA axis: A comprehensive review. Int. J. Mol. Sc. 18: 1687 pp 1- 14

The use of dentures in older people with low numbers of teeth greatly improves chewing and is accompanied by increased masticatory muscle activity and occlusal force as well as demonstrable prefrontal brain activity.

Some manufacturers have now created non-toxic 'chewing toys' for children with problems like autism or older adults with declining brain function to allow them to stimulate their brains through chewing. Chewing non-sugar gum is highly recommended for anyone who is more capable. Mastication can improve some aspects of brain performance such as working memory and alertness and considerably reduce depression and anxiety.

Watch and copy?

Researchers in this field are also hampered by the loss of interest in chewing in people who are already suffering from dementia. Some researchers are trying to evoke 'copying' by using the dining rooms of dementia patients to show videos of people chewing. The results are not yet available. It could well be too late for these people, but this work shows us that good nutrition alone is insufficient to keep us well.

Eye health and aging

Eyes are also affected by age and apart from presbyopia – the loss of the ability to focus at very close objects, which is usually obvious at about age 40, the other three problems can be very serious and lead to blindness if not treated appropriately.

As well as age itself, most eye conditions are influenced by a person's genes and most can also be induced by (a) eye injury, (b) high blood pressure and (c) medications, especially corticosteroids. Poorly controlled blood sugar levels in diabetes can cause eye disease and smoking also increases the risk of macular degeneration.

The regular use of quality dark glasses to protect against ultraviolet light, wind and dust will reduce the risk of all eye problems. Furthermore, like almost every other aspect of health, a high-quality diet with all the necessary micronutrients will also protect the health of our eyes.

Three serious eye conditions are commonly found in older people and it is advisable to have an eye check-up at least once every two years to detect these in their earliest stages.

Macular degeneration

Age-related macular degeneration is the primary cause of irreversible blindness in people aged 65 and over living in developed countries. It is currently thought to affect between 30 and 50 million people and this number is growing rapidly. There are two forms of this disease called 'wet' and 'dry' and whilst there are no effective treatments currently available for the 'dry' form, the 'wet' form is treated by the injection of drugs into the eye.

Cataracts

Cataracts, which cause cloudy, double-vision and sensitivity to light are also increased with age, smoking, high blood sugar and too much direct eye exposure to sunlight.

Glaucoma

Like the other eye diseases associated with aging, Glaucoma, a change in the pressure inside the eye, whilst also increased by genetic predisposition is also increased by diabetes, heart disease, eye injury and medications.

Age-related Eye Problems:
Lutein, Zeaxanthin and Fish

The effects of diet on age-related eye diseases have been tested in many studies and these studies in turn have been assessed for quality and consistency in systematic reviews.

Two 'carotenoids' or groups of carotenoids called Lutein and Zeaxanthin, often referred to as L/Z are known to be essential for the maintenance of the pigment of the macular. The macular is a small spot near the center of the retina at the back of the eye that is essential for sharp vision focus and allows us to see objects that are straight ahead. Consequently, a good deal of research has examined the role of dietary L/Z in maintaining good macular function.

The following vegetables and fruits are rich sources of L/Z: kale, parsley, spinach, broccoli, peas, oranges, honeydew melon, kiwifruit, red peppers, squash and grapes. Ten of eleven studies showed a large reduction in risk of macular problems with increase in dietary L/Z. Only one study failed to show a statistically significant result but even this study showed a positive association. HOWEVER, the vegetables need to be eaten *with fat* to enable their absorption and the best fats to use are one or more of *egg yolk, olive oil* or *coconut oil.*

Diets that included eating fish about twice a week also seemed to be beneficial but like all health problems, a diet that is high in refined carbohydrates and fats and low in vitamins will ACCELERATE more rapid deterioration in eye health.

Chapter fifteen

OLIVES, OLIVE OIL & HEALTHY FATS

Mediterranean foods to the rescue

The 'Mediterranean Diet' is not a single diet but it does have some important elements. Regarding it as a single diet is a similar error to the extrapolations that led to the huge mistakes made in the research undertaken in the 1960's and 1970's. But it seems we don't learn and here for an example of a somewhat erroneous definition is one on the internet from the prestigious organization The Mayo Clinic. I have crossed out the errors! Canola oil does NOT replace Olive Oil.

*'The **Mediterranean diet** emphasizes: Eating primarily plant-based foods, such as fruits and vegetables, whole grains, legumes and nuts. ~~Replacing butter~~ with healthy fats such as olive oil and ~~canola~~ oil. Using herbs and spices instead of salt to flavor foods.'*

It is true that some regions of the Mediterranean eat many plant-based foods, but I doubt that many 'primarily' eat plant-based foods. and I doubt that <u>any</u> (at least traditionally) eat 'canola oil' so I have crossed that out. Also, although most, if not all Mediterranean people eat olive oil, there has been virtually no research conducted on the use of butter.

So, in protest I am going to refer to this quasi diet as a MD style of diet and then discuss the range of wonderful foods that are typical of this region.

Traditional Mediterranean Diets

One stable component of the Mediterranean is Olive Oil and not too surprisingly Olives. Olive trees grow extremely well in the Mediterranean climate and require very little irrigation, so it isn't surprising that the Mediterranean countries have used this as their staple. I have been lucky enough to have made many trips to Italy, Spain, Greece and France but one of the noticeable things about the food is that every small region has its own delicacies. As an example of the diversity, the next table shows the key ingredients common in the cuisines of three large regions of Spain.

We readily see that all three regions consume olive oil, garlic and onions, cheese and tomatoes but other vegetables vary and presumably reflect the foods that grow well in the local areas. All three regions also consume some seafood, but in two of the regions this is not primarily fish and includes more shellfish and foods such as eels that many of us might not have encountered. Eels, as it happens are an extremely nutritious food, but like many other healthy foods, they are becoming the victims of chemical pollution and are likely victims of climate change.

Cheese and dairy foods are hardly mentioned in the literature on the MD, but cheese and yoghurt are very important components of the diet in all Mediterranean countries, and throughout Europe are a key source of vitamin K2, which will be discussed further below.

Both Basque and Andalusia have their own specialist cheeses that are made from the milk of sheep, goat and less commonly cow's milk. Yoghurt and other fermented milk products are also commonly consumed.

REGION	MOST COMMON INGREDIENTS
BASQUE	Olive oil, garlic/onion/leeks, chilli, white wine vinegar Prawns, clams or mussels, fish, chorizo, ham/pork, eggs. Cheese. Tomatoes, mushrooms, potatoes, green/red peppers.
ANDALUSIA	Olive oil, garlic/onion, white wine vinegar, parsley. Nuts, chicken, ham, fish, kidneys, brain, pig, tripe, eggs. Cheese. Spinach, tomatoes, potatoes, pimento.
VALENCIA	Olive oil, garlic/onion, rice, parsley Mussels, prawns, eels, snails, chicken, eggs, Cheese. Lettuce, sea-kale, peas, beans, green olives, asparagus, pimento, tomato.

Grapes are also grown throughout the Mediterranean countries and wine, especially red wine, is consumed with main meals.

Despite the tendency of some researchers to group these countries as if they are very similar, not only is each of the Mediterranean countries very distinctive but each has its own customs and cuisine. Indeed, there are really such big differences not only between countries but also between the regions within each country (for historical reasons) that a visitor might not even see much similarity.

What does stand out to the tourist, however, is the importance of the quality and freshness of the fruit and vegetables. Don't ever, as I have done, make the mistake of picking up a piece of fruit or vegetable in an Italian or French market – you will be in serious trouble! In all Mediterranean countries the fresh produce is highly valued and cared for in a manner that is extremely different from countries like Australia, Britain and the United States.

Olives and Olive Oil

The importance of Olive Oil lies in its major component Oleic Acid, which is **a critical unsaturated fatty acid that is a major component of all cellular and organelle membranes.** Since these membranes ultimately control almost all the functions of your body, it is critical that they become your number one health priority!

The oleic acid component of membranes is decreased by aging. **There is only one solution and it is an easy one – consume olive oil.**

Dr Shigeaki Hinohara, a Japanese doctor who died recently aged 105, was working 18 hours a day and walking up the stairs two at a time not long before his death. He had a simple diet but consumed **a tablespoon of olive oil** in orange juice for breakfast **every morning.**

I personally find it more palatable to pour my olive oil over my vegetables each evening but regardless of your approach, I think it is good to consume about a tablespoon of *room temperature* (raw) Extra Virgin Olive Oil every day.

Olive Oil isn't a very good oil for cooking at high temperatures because it has a lower smoke point than some other oils. This doesn't mean it isn't a good oil for cooking but if you want to cook something at very high temperature then you will be better off using oils like Safflower or Peanut Oil.

But as well as Oleic Acid, Olives also contain substances known as *Phenolics,* which are also found in many other plant foods. Phenolics have a range of complicated functions that assist our cells to function better. So, as well as having a high content of Oleic Acid, consuming Olive Oil will also give you a high intake of Phenolic compounds.

Drinks that are particularly high in phenolics include red wine, coffee and green tea and all the long-lived people <u>consumed at least one of these drinks every day.</u>

Cheese

We are aware that cheese is not only an important food throughout
Europe but that there are an extraordinarily large number of difference
cheeses, especially in France. These are not manufactured/processed
cheeses like many we see in our supermarkets, but each cheese has its
own very specific recipe that involves (a) the source of milk (type of
animal and perhaps specific pasture that the animal grazes on) (b) how it
is fermented and which strains of which bacteria and sometimes fungi
are used and (c) the exact conditions and time i.e. number of weeks of
fermentation.

With the recent understanding that there is a Vitamin called K2 that
plays a critical role in promoting both bone and cardiovascular health, it
was pleasing to find a publication that showed the results of analyses of
the long chain K2 content of several cheeses[32].

There may well be differences between the various manufacturers of the
same type of cheese, but I have created a Table from this publication
that gives the relative amounts of K2 present in some different cheeses.
Hopefully one day the labels on the cheeses will give us the K1 and K2
content so we know just how much we need to eat to reach our desired
value. Nevertheless, the K2 is created by the particular organism used in
the fermentation process and we should be able to assume that cheeses
of the same style have roughly the same K2 content.

[32] Vermeer C et al (2018) Menaquinone content of cheese. Nutrients 10: 446; doi:
10.3390/nu10040446

Although short chain K2 (known as Phylloquinone) as found in Kimchee is clearly very effective given that the South Koreans have the world's lowest level of deaths from cardiovascular disease, this must be eaten every day and some publications suggest that it isn't as effective as Menaquinone, which is the name of the long chain K2 that lasts longer in our bodies. All fermented cheeses show some increased values of menaquinone after more weeks of ripening until they reach a plateau, where the level remains stable. The next Table shows some total vitamin K2 levels ng/gm for some well-known cheeses. In general, Italian cheeses are quite low in K2 and overall medium to soft cheeses have more K2 than hard cheeses.

Cheese	Country of Origin	Total K2 (ng/gm)
Gouda (13 weeks)	Netherlands	656
Maasdam (5 weeks)	Netherlands	647
Brie	France	125
Camembert	France	681
Münster	France	801
Feta	Greece	117
Gorgonzola	Italy	153
Pecorino	Italy	94
Emmenthal	Switzerland	433
Gruyere	Switzerland	65
Gamalost	Norway	542

Another recent paper reports that multiple forms of Vitamin K also exist in other dairy foods but especially in Yoghurt[33] made from full cream milk. There was little difference between Greek and regular yoghurt but <u>neither</u> had <u>any</u> K2 if they were produced from skim (fat free) milk.

And before I leave K2, there is compelling data that vitamin K2 and Vitamin D work in synergy to stabilize both bones and the vessels of the cardiovascular system as well as improving dental health.

I personally believe that Cod Liver Oil, which contains both Vitamin A and D is a very safe and beneficial source of each of these vitamins. Some medical literature is concerned about possible Vitamin A toxicity and promotes the less effective source of beta carotene, but it takes a huge amount of Vitamin A for toxicity and in my own experience a daily capsule of Cod Liver Oil causes no problems. Its role is to help maintain the health of all your epithelial cells – the cells that form all your outside and inside 'linings'.

Garlic and Onion

It is very noticeable just how much garlic is used in Spanish cooking. Both garlic and onion are used in most Mediterranean dishes but generally it isn't such a standout as it is in Spain. Garlic and onion will be discussed in the next chapter about the importance of consuming sulfur in your diet.

---

[33] Fu X, Harshman SG, Shen X et al (2017) Multiple Vitamin K forms exist in dairy foods. Current developments in Nutrition 1:e000638

Other healthy fats affected by aging

Gamma linolenic acid (GLA)

When I first looked at the data on fatty acids in adipose tissue samples from the Scottish Heart study, the fatty acid whose decline really stood out was Gamma-linolenic Acid (GLA). This indeed was the greatest change observed in any fatty acid for both males and females. The starting and finishing values were greater (about double) in males than females but in both men and women, and between the average ages of 42 and 57, GLA levels had declined 9.3% in men and 17.6% in women (shown in the Figure below). Presumably these levels continue to decline throughout the remainder of life.

A big problem with this decline is that there are no simple foods sources of GLA and <u>once you are aging, no other dietary fatty acids will convert into it</u>. So, GLA needs to be supplemented and as far as I know there are only three reliable natural sources, namely Borage seed oil, Blackcurrent seed oil and Evening Primrose seed oil. GLA is also found in varying amounts in edible **hemp** seeds, oats, barley, and **spirulina.**

When you are younger, you can convert linoleic acid into GLA but the enzyme that performs this reaction is progressively shut down with aging. GLA supplementation probably won't benefit anyone under about 35 because it is only at about age 40 that our own ability to metabolize fatty acids really declines.

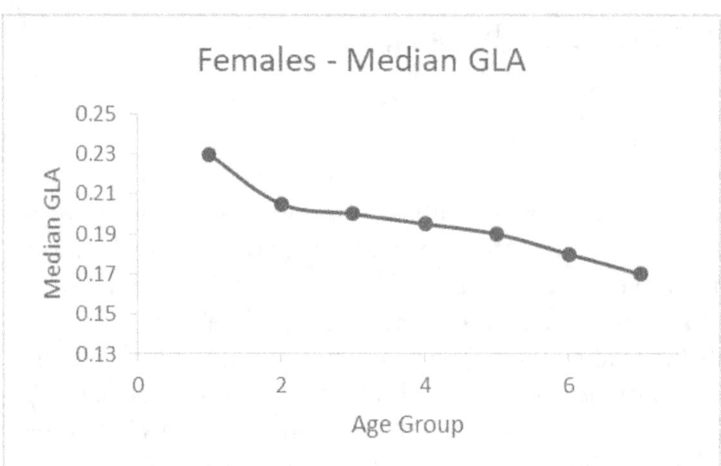

Figure: median values of gamma linolenic acid in adipose tissue in women in the Scottish Heart Study. Age groups are: 1 = 25-30, 2 = 31-33. 3 = 34-36, 4 = 37-39, 5 = 40-42, 5 = 43-45, 6 = 46-49.

Borage officinalis is an herb that grows as a common weed in the Mediterranean countries. The seeds contain about 26% gamma linolenic acid (GLA). Similarly, another weedy plant *Oenothera biennis* – known as *Evening Primrose Oil* originated in the central states of North America and the plant was used for healing by the indigenous tribes of the region. Its seeds contain about 24% GLA and it is more commonly used as a source of GLA but most of the available supplements only contain 10% GLA.

Both plants are easy to cultivate in a home garden but if you decide to grow your own source of GLA, (Oenothera) Evening Primrose is the safer option as all parts of the plant can be consumed if desired.

GLA & INFLAMMATION

Many scientific studies have demonstrated that diets supplemented with GLA have reduced levels of inflammation. GLA plays an important role in modulating inflammation throughout the body and is incorporated into the membranes of immune system cells. Recent studies have demonstrated that it reduces chronic inflammation in general but specifically eczema, dermatitis, asthma, rheumatoid arthritis, atherosclerosis, diabetes, obesity and even some forms of cancer.

For the few of you who would like the scientific explanation: GLA regulates the inflammatory "master molecule" *nuclear factor-kappa B or NF-kB* and prevents it from switching on genes for inflammatory cytokines in cell nuclei. Also, like some of the other beneficial fatty acids, GLA also activates the extremely powerful peroxisome proliferator-activated receptor *(PPAR)* system. PPARs are intracellular receptors that modulate cell metabolism and responses to inflammation.

GLA & DIABETES

GLA supplementation can play a therapeutic role in type 2 diabetes. One recent study of females aged between about 50 and 60, who all had either metabolic syndrome or early stage type 2 diabetes, found that eight weeks supplementation with GLA significantly lowered total and low-density cholesterol whereas the control group taking corn oil showed no changes.

Diabetes is often associated with nerve damage *neuropathy* and an **itching** disorder called *neurodermatitis* that can be a very unpleasant, tormenting side effect. Several scientific studies and review articles show that GLA can gradually reduce these effects without interfering with any of the drugs controlling glucose levels. Please don't expect an overnight cure!

GLA AND ATHEROSCLEROSIS

One of the key roles of vitamin K2 is ameliorating atherosclerosis by moving calcium out of the blood vessels and into bones and teeth, where it belongs. But another factor in the development of atherosclerosis is inflammation and the inflammation can be greatly reduced with the use of GLA (as well as by the key enzymes discussed earlier) .

I mentioned above that when GLA is taken up by the membranes of immune cells, it modulates their function. So, by the same mechanism GLA is incorporated into platelets and it reduces their tendency to clump together within small blood vessels. So GLA supplementation will also reduce the risk of stroke and heart attacks.

Palmitoleic, Linoleic and eicosenoic acids

In the Scottish Heart Study, only three other fatty acids were reduced by aging and these can all be obtained quite easily from foods. Linoleic acid is found in most if not all nuts and seeds so we should certainly increase our intake of these as we age to compensate for the reductions that occur as a function of aging. Eicosenoic acid is found in peanut oil, butter and other fats but its levels are only minimally influenced by aging because of its ready availability in most diets.

Little research has been performed on palmitoleic acid, which is an omega 7 fatty acid, present in macadamia nuts and is reduced in aging. Most research suggests that although this is an unsaturated fatty acid, it behaves like a saturated fatty acid and may not have any health benefits?

The Internet and Medical Literature are both full of claims about fish oil but some of this is probably quite misguided. I understand that fish oil was originally trialed as a treatment for rheumatoid arthritis (RA) because it reduced inflammation by competing with arachidonic acid. Fish oil had some benefits for RA but this is not the same disease – nor is it related in any way except by age to osteoarthritis!

Data on Fatty acids in adipose tissue in the Scottish Heart Study showed that the long chain Omega 3 fatty acids were slightly *increased* with age, rather than decreased like all others. This is probably because they are <u>very important</u> and when the whole system is compromised, they are 'preferred' rather than less important fatty acids. So, it is a good idea to have a regular intake of these fatty acids (probably as fish itself) but just how much is disputed. ALPHA LINOLEIC ACID (ALA) is often recommended as a healthy Omega 3 fatty acid. This is true but as you age your body will be <u>unable to convert</u> ALA to the longer chain fatty acids (DHA and EPA) found in fish and fish oil and so if you don't eat fish, you *should* supplement with some fish oil.

A couple of years ago I attended a scientific presentation where there was a huge difference in opinion on supplementation with fish oils. The presenter, a public health physician, claimed that eating fish twice a week gave an adequate intake whereas a physiologist in the audience was strongly disputing this and advocating daily supplementation. So, what is the real position?

A detailed publication from a group representing the American Heart Society recently reviewed the results of many huge studies (involving thousands of participants) on the use of fish oil in cardiovascular disease[34]. Their conclusions were that there was *very little evidence* that fish oil supplementation had any effect!

---

[34] Siscovick DS et al (2017) Omega-3 polyunsaturated fatty acid (fish oil) supplementation and the prevention of clinical Cardiovascular Disease. Circulation 135: e867-e884

Other studies show that fish oil supplementation *does not lower inflammation* as measured by C-reactive protein or interleukin-6 levels in healthy adults. Because of the general promotion for the advantages of fish oil, I was at first rather surprised by these negative results but in view of the functions of vitamin K2 and GLA, it's easy enough to see that many researchers have been heading in the wrong direction.

So, returning to the seminar, it seems that the public health physician seemed to know what she was talking about!

Are there any benefits of eating fish and/or taking fish oil?

Considering the media attention, generalized promotion and discussion of fish oil, there is very little evidence that it has major benefits in older adults beyond its content of *Vitamin D*. Many adults are deficient in this key vitamin and in times of low sun exposure – especially winter and especially in winter for people with darker skin, then some supplementation with Vitamin D is necessary. Again, I prefer Cod Liver Oil, because I think that we do need extra Vitamin A, but some others will not agree with this despite all the evidence!

Eating fish, especially wild fish if you can find it, is a good source of Selenium in addition to Vitamin D, Phosphorus and the Omega 3 fatty acids. Nevertheless, eating fish and shellfish is not without risk as they can be a source of mercury, allergens and several different biotoxins, some of which are lethal. Since you need to be VERY CAREFUL about the source of the fish you eat and its handling, eating high quality **tinned wild sardines** might in fact be the least expensive and safest option.

Chapter sixteen

SULFUR, MINERALS AND VITAMINS

Sulfur requirements & age-related deficiency

As we age, we require more sulfur both to accommodate our on-going whole of life sulfur requirements plus all the extra we require to support our most important enzyme **glutathione-S-tranferase** (GST) in its critical roles of detoxification, cellular storage and transport, regulation of cellular signalling and control of inflammation. Our need for this enzyme's help *increases with every year of aging* and the 'S' in GST stands for sulfur.

Without dietary sulfur for periods of 10 days, even young healthy 25 year old men halved their whole blood glutathione synthesis[35]. So, inadequate ongoing sulfur intake in older people can have devastating consequences.

Since sulfur is involved in so many critical cellular functions, deficiency can cause or exacerbate a wide range of symptoms. There are so many and they are so important that I am going to list several of them in categories:

---

[35] Lyons J et al (2000) Blood glutathione synthesis rates in healthy adults receiving a sulfur amino acid-free diet. Proceedings National Academy Science 97 (10): 5071-5076

- Epidermal (skin related): acne, brittle nails, hair loss (balding), rashes, slow wound healing
- Gastrointestinal: various
- Metabolic in general: obesity, insulin resistance, chronic fatigue
- Brain function: depression, memory loss, Alzheimer's, convulsions
- Joints: osteoarthritis and other symptoms of inflammation.

It doesn't seem to matter too much how you obtain your sulfur, but as I have mentioned several times already, sulfur is needed for the function of glutathione-S-transferase, which is your major detoxifying enzyme. As we age, more and more of our cells become senescent so the requirement for sulfur *continues to increase* throughout life.

Sulfur Cures in History and Balneotherapy

Sulfurous baths have been used for centuries, apparently to great benefit but like many other similar events they tend to have been accepted by the religious as miracles and rejected by conventional medicine and science. Fortunately, many people have continued to use them and now recent research has proven that there are real benefits.

A substantial amount of research has been undertaken to establish whether inorganic sulphate can actually be absorbed via the lungs and through the skin and two review articles conclude that this is so[36] [37]. Thus, while high levels of hydrogen sulphide (rotten egg gas) are extremely toxic, the body can easily detoxify low levels to organic sulphate and low levels can be tolerated indefinitely.

---

[36] Mitchell SC & Waring RH (2016) Sulphate absorption across biological membranes. Xenobiotica 46: 184-191.

[37] Carbajo JM & Maraver F (2017) Sulphurous Mineral Waters: New applications for health.

If you are one of the many aging people who is suffering from joint stiffness or any of the other problems listed above, then you need either take to the sulfur baths on a very regular basis or to add some sulfur to your diet. Interestingly, one research study conducted at a health resort on patients with chronic degenerative arthritis found that those who used sulfur baths for 3-weeks had very much better results than the age-matched group who used spa therapy for the same time. Not only did the sulfur group have a significant decline in all the infammatory markers but their cholesterol levels also improved.

Are the dietary recommendations for sulfur too low?

In a review article[38] on dietary sulfur, the authors point out that the calculations for daily dietary minimal recommendations for all the essential acids are based on their ability to maintain a suitable nitrogen balance. Since the sulfur content of the amino acids has been ignored in these calculations, the current estimations and recommendations could be quite unsuitable!

Despite sulfur being the third most abundant mineral in our bodies after calcium and phosphorus, only two of the 20 amino acids contain sulfur and one of these, methionine cannot be synthesized by us and therefore must be obtained from the diet. We can synthesise the second amino acid cysteine but this requires a steady supply of sulfur. So in addition to the aging body's high requirement for sulfur to support glutathione, it is generally in short supply in our diets.

Evidence-based Complimentary & Alternative Medicine Article ID 8034084

[38] Nimni ME et al (2007) Are we getting enough sulfur in our diet?

Nutrition & Metabolism 4: 24 - pp 1 -12, http://www.nutritionandmetabolism.com/contents/4/1/24

The (current) daily recommended amount of methionine can be fairly readily obtained by eating 100 gm of lean beef, lamb, turkey, chicken, pork, oily fish or two eggs. Vegetarians can obtain it in nuts, seeds and beans but they need to consume higher amounts. Nevertheless, I have always consumed about that amount of methionine-based foods and it hasn't been enough to sustain my hip cartilage. It may be, as Nimni says, that even though these recommendations are specifically for methionine that the amounts are still calculated for nitrogen rather than sulfur?

One effective way to supplement dietary sulfur is to drink sulfated water throughout the day. Sulfur is absorbed effectively this way but San Pellegrino is one of few Mineral Waters that reliably contains sulfur, and although pleasant enough, this might be an expensive way of obtaining sufficient sulfur. You will no doubt think though – ah, yes, here is something that many Mediterraneans do that hasn't been listed as part of the Mediterranean diet!

Common drugs deplete sulfur!

Do you ever take the drug which is called one of these names: paracetamol/tylenol/acetaminophen, for minor pain? If you are having some joint pain you are likely to this and sadly, *ultimately* this will make your pain much worse! Drugs like acetaminophen require large amounts of sulfur for their excretion.

A toxic metabolite of acetaminophen called N-acetyl-p-benzoquinoneimine is detoxified by hepatic glutathione. If you take acetaminophen, you literally use up more glutathione detoxifying the drug that you used to eliminate the pain caused by the sulfur deficiency!

Other forms of dietary sulfur and supplements

The Allium family of plants includes many tasty nutritious vegetables that are each a rich source of sulfur. These include onion, garlic, scallion, shallot, leek and chives and as you know, if they are used judiciously, they add great flavour to foods. Other vegetables like broccoli and brussels sprouts have much lower levels.

Sadly, many people can't eat any of the Allium vegetables, or only in very small quantities, because they all contain quite high amounts of long-chain polysaccharides called fructans. Many people can only tolerate tiny amounts of fructans because they cause them painful bloating and diarrhoea. If you, like me are one of these people, you may need to take some type of sulfur supplement to consume adequate sulfur. Supplementation could be necessary once you reach about age 50 so if possible, start supplementing before you get problems.

Chondroitin and glucosamine are offered as pharmaceutical sources of sulfur, especially for arthritis or joint problems and other sulfur compounds such as SAMe, DMSO and reduced glutathione are all used as drugs to restore sulfur metabolism.

I developed debilitating arthritis of both hips in 2003 and tried taking three of the four supplements above without any noticeable relief. One pharmacy introduced me to a combined powder that included MSM, a form of organic sulfur (methylsulfoxymethane) and I had a remarkable reduction in the level of discomfort. Later, I discovered an inexpensive source of pure MSM and found that it not only worked better for me than the mixture but that it is also inexpensive.

My hips had deteriorated too much to be restored by sulfur so I had two hip replacements in 2009. But I continue to take my MSM and I just sprinkle about one teaspoon on my breakfast each day. I have never experienced any negative side effects from it.

When I started taking MSM in about 2008, when it wasn't well known, I was told that it worked as an analgesic. But while it certainly did reduce pain, it also seemed to gradually improve my joint function. This is clearly because it is a very effective source of sulfur.

MSM is now quite widely used and may be called 'dimethyl sulfone', 'methyl sulfone', sulfonylbismethane, organic sulfur or crystalline dimethyl sulfoxide. Regardless of what it is called, MSM acts as a sulfur donor. It is readily absorbed and seems to be completely safe.

Recent research suggests that MSM's function is likely to be influenced by a person's microbiome so at least at the start, one person might find it more effective than another. The great thing about consuming sulfur is that it improves all your issues at once. All the problems that were listed at the beginning of this chapter - skin, nails, allergies, gut, fatigue, brain as well as joints – are all improved by enough sulfur.

Other Minerals and Vitamins

I have already discussed vitamin K2 extensively and how it works synergistically with Vitamins A and D. Vitamins C and E also seem to be involved in enhancing the health of the endothelial cells that line the arteries. Both C and E are powerful antioxidants and can help our bodies clean up the superoxide anions and other reactive oxygen-derived species that are produced by the ever-growing number of senescent cells that are produced by aging.

Vitamin D is one of the vitamins that is frequently deficient and whose deficiency increases the risk of a range of problems from depression to obesity, diabetes and hypertension. I referred to Vitamin D intake in a previous chapter and recommended sunshine, where possible, or supplementation with Cod Liver Oil. Taking Cod Liver Oil also ensures that you have enough Vitamin A and although *excess* Vitamin A is toxic, a daily capsule of Cod Liver Oil is only a low dose. Vitamin A will improve your vision as well as supporting your immune system. As I commented earlier, deficiencies of Vitamin A affect the health of all your epithelial cells – the cells that form all your out

Recent studies have found that people with lower back pain are very likely to be vitamin D deficient, especially if the pain is severe. Low Vitamin D levels are also found in association with bone fractures and if the Vitamin D deficiency is severe, this can cause secondary Hyperparathyroidism and related hip fractures. It is important that both Calcium intake and Vitamin D levels are adequate.

Earlier I discussed the latest research that suggests that Alzheimer's Disease is associated with a disturbance of copper metabolism. The literature on this topic seems to be somewhat inconsistent, but the latest data shows that people with Alzheimer's have lower than normal levels of copper in their brains and higher levels in their blood cells. In other words, there appears to be a disruption of copper control mechanisms that might be caused by higher than normal exposures to copper and/or other factors that affect copper metabolism?

A recent review of research related to Vitamins in Alzheimer's Disease[39] showed that B vitamins are involved as co-factors in all the core biochemical pathways. Moreover, low blood concentrations of Vitamins A, B-12, C, E and Folic Acid are consistently found in the blood of Alzheimer's patients and these vitamins as well as dietary unsaturated fatty acids play protective roles against dementia.

Iodine and thyroid health

Our thyroid gland, a small gland in the neck is our key metabolic and temperature regulator. I first 'confronted' the thyroid when a woman, who was seeking my advice regarding her infertility, arrived on a warm day, wearing a heavy coat. I don't think I had seen a goiter before, but I knew what it was immediately. The very sad thing was that this woman had been receiving quite intense psychiatric care and her obvious goiter hadn't been detected!

We had a specialist thyroid clinic at the hospital where I was working and so I called them for advice on how to confirm my 'diagnosis' and was told how to conduct a 'heel reflex' test. The reflex was absent in my visitor and so I sent her off to receive care for her thyroid. I was delighted when about six months later, she called in to thank me – goiter gone, slim, healthy and almost unrecognizable.

After that occasion I came across many other undiagnosed thyroid cases. One, a family who had (completely overlooked) familial hypothyroidism – Hashimoto's thyroiditis – had several adults both male and female who were infertile and one seriously retarded child who had been hypothyroid from birth and institutionalized. A second child in the family had died at about age four.

An underactive thyroid can't maintain body temperature and apart from causing weight gain and infertility, is a major cause of depression. Sometimes it is caused by Hashimoto's, which is a dominant gene so passes from a parent directly to child. Like all dominant genes it has variable expression, so a child can express the gene more strongly than a parent and females often express this gene more than males.

---

[39] Fenech M (2017) Vitamins associated with brain aging. Mild cognitive impairment, and Alzheimer Disease. Thematic Review Series: 4th International Vitamin Conference. Advances in Nutrition 8: 958-970.

But hypothyroidism isn't always genetic and is frequently caused by iodine deficiency. A friend and colleague, Basil Hetzel, who died a few years ago, spent his life trying to defeat worldwide thyroid illness caused by low dietary intake of Iodine. He succeeded in having Iodine added to salt but sadly much of the recent advice to reduce salt, plus 'fashions' in salt, have meant that many people are (again) now iodine deficient.

Seaweed is a very good source of dietary iodine, but it is reasonably easy to overdose and develop some symptoms of hyperthyroidism, which I describe below. I think that my current intake of **two kelp-wrapped sushi** each week is about the right amount, but you might find that you might need a little more at the beginning if you start off with low levels of iodine?

Hyperthyroidism

Hyperthyroidism is less common than hypothyroidism but its most common cause is called Graves' Disease. This is an autoimmune condition in which the immune cells inappropriately start producing antibodies that stimulate the thyroid to overproduce thyroid hormone. People with this condition often develop bulging eyes but the common symptoms are racing heart, shaky hands, difficulty sleeping, weight loss, muscle weakness, heat intolerance and neuropsychiatric symptoms.

Mineral intake and phytic acid

Phytic acid is the major storage form of phosphorus in cereals, legumes, oil seeds and nuts and humans don't have the ability to break it down. It is found at varying concentrations in these foods with the highest levels in cereal bran and seeds such as linseed, sesame seed and sunflower meal. There can be quite a range in different products with walnuts, for example, ranging from 0.20 to 6.69 gm per 100 gm by dry weight!

Unfortunately, phytic acid greatly reduces the potential value of diets that are rich in these foods because it acts as an *anti-nutritive agent* by blocking the absorption of minerals such as iron, zinc, magnesium, manganese, selenium and calcium, <u>which then all pass out in the feces</u>.

Phytic acid can be removed by fermentation, soaking and germination and this is one major reason why these traditional forms of food preparation have such beneficial effects. Fermentation might take some skills but soaking nuts and seeds and either drying them in the sun, in a low temperature oven or a dryer are relatively easy and effective ways of greatly increasing the nutrition you can obtain from all the cereals, legumes, oilseeds and nuts that you consume. Do make sure that your drying methods are effective, or your foods will grow fungi, which will be worse for you than the phytic acid!

Nevertheless, if you eat a diet that is rich in these foods and you don't eliminate the phytic acid, you may still need to take supplements to receive adequate intakes of minerals.

How do you know if you need to take supplements?

The whole area of nutrition, vitamins and minerals is extremely complex and outside the scope of this book. Laboratory tests are often helpful but even chemical analyses of different types of tissues – blood, adipose, hair and/or nails will only give you a picture and not necessarily a diagnosis.

Self-reflection and self-evaluation are probably the best tools for detecting deficiencies and these used to be the ordinary things that doctors, chemists and our mothers used to check. You can start by checking these yourself and if you are not sure what is normal, consult some of the large number of resources on the Internet.

- Do your finger and toenails grow normally and are they strong? Do they have any unusual ridges and/or spots or anything worse?
- Do you have a clean, pink tongue?
- Are your gums clean, pink and intact? They should not bleed when you clean your teeth.
- Is your hair strong or does it split?
- Do you sleep well most nights? Do you ever suffer from 'restless legs'? If so, magnesium supplements might reduce this symptom as well as enhancing your sleep quality.
- Do you have good color in your face and are the whites of your eyes 'white'?
- Do you feel more tired than is justified by your level of activity? Do you have energy appropriate for your age? Please aim to be better than expected for your age!
- Do you suffer from cramps?
- Are you depressed?

Unfortunately, many older people are given ongoing medications that either restrict their dietary vitamins or cause vitamin deficiencies. I am going to give one example here, which is quite a common problem but there are many others.

Vitamin B12 (cobalamin) is essential to normal brain function. Deficiency in B12 not only causes the brain to malfunction but it also causes structural damage to the brain so that a range of abnormal neuropsychiatric symptoms can develop via disturbances in different parts of the brain.[40]

Despite its availability in common foods, B12 deficiency is frequently found in older adults. The estimates of deficiency range from 3% to 40%, with the higher rates mostly occurring in institutional settings. B12 is one of the most readily available vitamins in an omnivorous diet as it is in rich supply in dairy foods, eggs, beef and lamb – and especially in any organ meats and in all oily fish. Many cereals and soy products are fortified with B12 so that vegetarians can also easily access the vitamin.

In some cases, deficiencies are caused by poor diets, but other factors and conditions frequently interfere with its appropriate absorption. These are listed as:

- Atrophic gastritis – commonly caused by a long-term infection with *Helicobacter pylori* and sometimes by an autoimmune condition.
- Chronic gastritis – this has several causes, including age itself but it can be induced by over-use of everyday pain relievers aspirin, ibuprofen or naproxen.
- Drug interactions including metformin or one of many other commonly prescribed drugs that can increase gastric pH such as histamine 2 blockers, proton pump inhibitors (PPIs), colchicine (for gout), cholestyramine, anticonvulsants,

[40] Lachner C et al (2019) The neuropsychiatry of Vitamin B12 deficiency in elderly patients. J. Neuropsychiatry. https://doi.org/10.1176/appi.neuopsych.11020052

antibiotics, nitrous oxide and antacids. Various drugs can also lead to bacterial overgrowth of the small intestine, which is common in elderly people and this may also increase B12 deficiency.

- Several medical conditions including pernicious anemia and Sjorgren's syndrome, chronic pancreatitis, Crohn's disease, Whipple's disease, celiac disease, amyloidosis, scleroderma, intestinal lymphomas or tuberculosis.
- Surgical procedures on the gut

If you have experienced or are experiencing any of these conditions, or taking any of the many relevant drugs, it is likely that you will probably need to take vitamin supplements and/or eat more of some types of foods.

Unfortunately, many drugs prevent you from consuming nutrient rich foods, so it is important that you have an in-depth conversation with your doctor about the need for you to take a drug or undertake a procedure. You also need to know whether it will be necessary or possible for you to take supplements to compensate for any ill effects?

Fruit and vegetables – obtaining a 'fresh' supply!

High quality fresh fruit and vegetables are full of nutrients, but the levels decline quite quickly once they are harvested and transported. The best of all possible options is to grow your own vegetables, but this isn't possible for most people. The next option is to buy seasonal fruit and vegetables that have been grown as close to where you live as possible. Farmers' markets are usually great places to buy your produce.

Once the produce has been harvested, levels of nutrients start declining and so the time taken in transport and then in shelf display, will mean that the nutrients have reduced long before you get the produce home. If you live a long distance from where the produce is grown you are probably much better off purchasing frozen, canned or dried food because this will be far more nutritious.

If you can buy fresh fruit and vegetables, then the general rules are:

- Put all the produce in the refrigerator, except tomatoes, unripe avocados and root vegetables, as soon as you get home.
- Don't wash or cut the produce until you are ready to cook it or to eat it raw.
- Cook minimally. Steaming preserves more nutrients than any other form of cooking.
- If you are intending to store your produce in the refrigerator, only buy enough for one week's consumption.
- Try to eat a variety of different colored fruits and vegetables. This will give you a much greater range of nutrients than larger servings of a few vegetables.

Heat, light and oxygen all reduce the nutrients in fruit and vegetables so remember this when you are transporting your produce between the shop and home. If you have several errands to perform, leave your food shopping till last to maximize the nutrients that you will eventually consume.

Chapter seventeen

BODY AND MIND EXERCISE & AGING WELL

Your Exercise Regimes

Your personality and your exercise regimes

Unlike the previous chapters where I have referred extensively to the medical and scientific literature, here I am just speaking from my own experience and the advice I have received from a large variety of sources throughout my life. I do think that everyone needs to exercise but I don't think that the same types of exercise suit everyone. Moreover, I believe that although some regimes are primarily physical and some are primarily mental, we need to consider and undertake some of each type.

Types of exercise for 'the body'

If we think about exercise for the body, we can immediately see that there are many different aspects to this.

One important consideration is the levels of interaction you might make with others whilst undertaking the exercises. In general, performing precisely the same exercise alone will not be the same experience as performing it in a group or in the presence of other people. In general, time goes faster and you can do more when you are not alone ....as long as you aren't distracted from the exercise!

I used to attend a variety of high intensity aerobic exercise classes some of which involved riding bikes, working out on different pieces of equipment, using hand weights and steps and most of these classes were accompanied by rousing music and ongoing encouragement from the instructor. I attended these classes when I travelled as well as at home and I was stunned when one American instructor asked me why I was training so hard? He said I was working too hard and should reduce my level unless I was training for a special event. But these types of classes encouraged competition and we enjoyed the competitive aspects. We sweated a great deal and we were extremely fit.

I do think that upbeat music on its own will inspire most people to work out harder in a gym but there is no doubt that – for most of us - being surrounded by others who are also working hard, makes the task easier.

Sport and exercise

There is really a fairly small distinction of considerable overlap between activities that are regarded as 'sports', which of course includes exercise versus those that are just regarded as 'exercise'. I suspect that calling something a sport usually implies that there is a competitive element although there are also (perhaps unspoken) competitive elements in all group exercise.

There are as many sports as there are different types of exercises, but for most people participating in sports or group exercise is much more beneficial in the long term than individual exercise. Whenever you participate in some type of sport, you are immediately encouraged to set goals. Provided these are both realistic and appropriate for you, you are very likely to keep participating in the activity and enjoy the personal challenge of trying to improve.

A well-organized group exercise session will have many similar benefits. You will have a social element that will usually encourage you to keep coming back and it will also tend to distract you from the 'pain' of exercise, so you will work harder for longer.

Individual training at a gym is easier to maintain than just performing exercises at home. Even so, exercising alone at a gym is not an easy thing to do and I wouldn't recommend it to beginners. In the first place you need to have a reasonable amount of experience to be able to use different pieces of equipment properly and you also need to have some guidance on which exercises are appropriate for you and how you should execute them. If you've had considerable advice and experience, then you certainly can work out on your own, but most people need to have quite a <u>specific routine</u> – the day and time when they go to the gym and what they do once they are there – or it is extremely easy to give up going. You don't mean to give up; it just happens!

Sport versus 'gym' and the range of 'functions' that are stimulated

I've spent a great deal of time playing sport but particularly tennis, then squash and now golf. There are obvious differences between the benefits offered by different sports e.g. tennis and (especially) squash use your reflexes much more than golf. However, most sports do much more than just exercise your body and is why I would recommend participating in sport in addition to exercising.

The following list identifies the quite large range of *physical and mental benefits* that you should seek to obtain through exercise and/or sport:

- *Focus and concentration:* Some is involved in exercising properly but probably not nearly as much is required as watching that ball till the very last second when it connects to your racquet, bat or golf club.

- *Muscular strength* is best developed in the gym (as well as for sport) because sport alone often develops muscles unevenly or fails to develop all the muscular strength that is really required. You need to strengthen all your muscles and so although aerobic exercise that primarily exercises your lower limbs and respiratory system is critical, everyone needs to work with weights to develop all the other muscles. It has been shown that high numbers of repetitions with light weights have much the same effects as fewer repetitions with heavier weights, so you don't have to be strong to undertake a weights-based program.

- *Core strength* is best developed in the gym or in Yoga and Pilates or equivalent classes. Having strong core muscles is essential to the function of your internal organs as well as your back.

- *Aerobic fitness:* If you walk the 18 holes of a golf course a couple of times a week or play some energetic games of tennis, you might receive enough exercise without also going to the gym, but this really depends on what you do in the time in between? If the rest of your time is spent sitting down, then you are probably not exercising enough.

Obviously, your health will determine just how much exercise you can do but most people can at least walk on a 'walking machine', ride a stationary bike or use a rowing machine. These machines in gyms can be set at levels where even the very elderly can work out effectively and 'aquarobics' is another safe exercise venue for those who have even very restricted abilities. But don't underestimate how hard you might work in an aquarobics class!

- *Sustained energy* is used in both sports and gym-based exercises but unless you are supervised or have some type of monitoring system (personal goals or 'apps'), sustained energy is usually more easily maintained while playing a sport.

- *Reflexes* are not often tested in a gym unless you are specifically working on this with a trainer. But it is very important that your reflexes are stimulated in some way. *Juggling* is one of the best and safe ways of stimulating reflexes and your reaction time and it's easy to obtain small, 'bean-bag' type juggling 'balls' in gift shops or online. Of course, in theory you can juggle anything, but these soft balls are easy to manage.

- *Balance* is frequently reduced with age and contributes to 'falls'. Balance is exercised a little in most sports, but this really needs active practice. *Tai Chi* is a wonderful exercise for building strength and endurance even in the very old. There are many videos available to help you but working with an experienced teacher in a group is extremely worthwhile. Tai Chi will also strengthen your core muscles as well as soothe your 'soul'.

- *Co-ordination and timing* are also improved by activities such as Tai Chi but all sports that involve hitting, catching, throwing/releasing (as in bowling) and/or kicking a ball or another device require high levels of hand and eye co-ordination. Many people find it much easier to hit and/or catch an object that is already moving than to hit a still object like a golf ball. This might be because reflexes are often better developed than concentration and this quite subtle difference in ability emphasizes the need for us to understand and practice each of these skills.

- *Fine motor skills and visual judgement* are important skills that are frequently required in everyday activities as well as in sport and can easily be compromised by illness. In golf, this is particularly used in putting but in everyday life these skills are used repeatedly in many activities including those as necessary as preparing food. Creative tasks such as sewing and knitting require high levels of fine motor skills and visual judgement, as do carpentry and similar activities. The introduction of 'men's sheds' has been very beneficial to older men's communication and comradery, but they have also enhanced or helped retain older men's fine motor skills.

- *Flexibility* is lost progressively with age from birth onwards! We just need to compare our older selves to a new baby to see just how rigid we become. Of course, some of this increased rigidity is associated with gains in muscle strength but Olympic gymnasts and dancers demonstrate that both power and flexibility can co-exist – but usually with an enormous amount of training!

Brain stimulation and training

Many of the activities, particularly sports I've listed above will stimulate your brain to some extent. You might have to keep and/or calculate scores. You often need to make complex judgements about speed, distance, height and angles and allow for factors like slope and wind and although many of these judgements are made subconsciously, they are still working your mind and your memory. But beyond this, it is desirable to continuously challenge your mind.

Many older people who live near me play Contract Bridge as an enjoyable past-time and brain stimulant, but I feel that Bridge may be a little too 'regimented' for me and involve too many hours of sitting? I have always loved 'reading' (especially novels) so I find that being a member of a relatively serious book club, where I prepare a detailed answer to a question on the monthly book, is an interesting activity.

But my aging brain probably needs still more challenges so beyond reading and spending some time thinking about 'science', I like to play a few different puzzles online each day. I usually play one or two games of easy or medium level *Sudoku* or two or three games of *Solitaire* and complete two on-line *Jigsaw* puzzles. Your choices in activities might be different to mine but crosswords, word challenges and other puzzles are all fun to do and very good for keeping our minds stimulated.

The Challenge of a new activity

Learning something that is completely new to you is not only engaging but energizing and is recommended for brain stimulation. Some suggest that we should adopt *at least one completely new activity every year of our lives*. Just about anything and everything will stimulate your brain and increase the enjoyment in your life.

There are endless number of activities, but a few suggestions are:

- Join a choir,
- Learn to play an instrument such as the Ukulele,
- Write a children's book,
- Take up photography,
- Learn another language – (probably the best)

Some activities will stimulate your brain and expand your life more than others but before you choose your next challenge, perhaps think about what is currently limiting your life and whether this new activity will satisfy a current unmet need or desire?

New activities will also usually introduce you to new people and this in turn could enrich your life in many unexpected ways.

Chapter eighteen

STRESS AND SLEEP

"When I look back on all these worries, I remember the story of the old man who said on his deathbed that he had had a lot of trouble in his life, most of which had never happened".

Winston Churchill

Like Winston Churchill, when we think about stress, we almost always think about psychological and emotional stress. But although emotional stress is foremost in our minds, it's probably not the stress our bodies evolved to face. Rather, our body's primary major stress response is a 'fight or flight' hormone called cortisol and clearly this stress response evolved in humans as it did in other animals to allow us to escape from physical danger.

It's easy to see that cortisol's actions are extremely helpful at times when we need to escape from marauding packs of lions or (occasionally) leap out of burning buildings. Cortisol diverts blood to our muscles, stimulates the production of glucose to give us more energy and shuts down our immune system, which is an unecessary 'luxury' at a time of crisis.

However, in modern life this adrenal-based system is often more of a hindrance than a help because most of the stress we suffer is of a psychological nature and the physical-based system can often work against us rather than for us.

Stress is complicated and the more it's studied the more complicated it seems to be. In a recent review the authors stated '*There seems to be no single definition that adequately describes stress* '[41].

Stress responses activate a link between the parts of the brain known as the hypothalamus and the pituitary and the adrenal gland (or HPA axis) and the part of the nervous system known as the sympathetic nervous system. This response can lead to many different biochemical changes throughout the entire body. Different types of stressors give rise to different patterns of response and it's more than likely that different individuals respond differently to similar stressors.

Stress and infection

There is a vast amount of data that proves that stress responses can suppress the immune system. This suppression seems to be able to occur almost immediately such that if, for example, soon after you have become stressed you happen to be close to a person with a 'contagious' illness, you are more likely to become infected. I have experienced this at least twice in the last 18 years (so not often) but it is extremely annoying when it happens.

---

[41] Pruett SB (2003) Stress and the immune system. Pathophysiology 9: 133-153

Deliberately putting yourself under enormous physical stress such as completely an ironman triathalon will overwhelm the immune system and it will remain depressed for three days or more afterwards, increasing an athlete's susceptibility to viral and bacterial infections. Triathletes generally understand these risks but people who are just pushing themselves past their usual limits are less likely to appreciate that they might also need to protect their immune systems for the next day or so.

Stress and risk of cancer

Links between stress and cancer have been suspected for a long time but it is a difficult area of research because the time between the stressful event/period and the diagnosis of the cancer can often be many years. Moreover since cancers grow at very different rates, setting parameters for investigations is very difficult. Nevertheless, as long ago as about the year 200 AD, Galen wrote that *melancholic* (i.e. emotionally sensitive and perfectionists) women were more susceptible to the 'swellings of the breast' than were *more sanguine* (i.e. more extroverted) women!

It is becoming more and more apparent that just the way you look at life can make a huge difference to your liklihood of experiencing a very large range of health issues!

Many studies in animals have also shown that stress can definitely affect the likelihood of a cancer *progressing.* One example in mice showed that in animals that were stressed by being confined in small spaces or isolated from other mice, existing tumors were more likely to grow and metastasize (spread) than in non-stressed mice with identical tumors. This effect of isolation could be very relevant to many people who feel isolated for a variety of reasons.

There are of course hundreds of published studies on this subject but one that I found helpful was a review of studies that addressed the 'psychological features of cancer'[42]. The problem is that chronic stress and depression lead to persistant activation of the HPA axis which suppresses parts of the immune system, in particular leads to decreased numbers of cytotoxic T-cells and natural-killer-cells. These cells usually conduct *immune surveillance* to detect and eliminate cancers and other mutated or genetically unstable cells.

Neurotransmitters, neurohormones and adrenal hormones all affect immune function because there are receptors for these 'cellular hormones' on the surfaces of immune cells like lymphocytes and macrophages.

Beyond the theory and the animal studies there is *clear evidence* that psychological and behavioural factors do affect the risk of having cancer and the risk of any cancer progressing. Nevertheless, it seems that not all cancer risks are equal and cancers that are induced by chemical carcinogens might be *less* affected by psychological, behavioural and immunological factors than those that are linked to *DNA viruses*. For example, most of us carry copies of Epstein Barr (EB) virus (the virus responsible for Glandular Fever), that are integrated into our DNA.

Suppression of our immune system can easily release this virus but this is usually associated with severe suppression of the immune system as might be seen in patients with AIDS or people with organ transplants.

---

[42] Reiche EDM et al (2004) Stress, depression, the immune system, and cancer. THE LANCET Oncology 5: 617-625

The brain-immune response can also work in the other direction. Because the interaction with the immune system involves most of the brain, as well as the brain affecting the immune system, illnesses that greatly activate the immune system (including trauma, sepsis and autoimmunity) can also cause mental disturbances. This isn't spoken about much and it's important to be aware that a person with an illness might be behaving oddly as a direct result of the illness and not just as a reaction to the discomfort the illness might be causing.

Minor discomforts induced by stress

Although relatively unimportant in the scheme of things, stress can induce discomfort that can still have a big impact on a person's life. I will list some of these:

- In susceptible people stress induced cortisol can cause diarrhoea because as well as the heart rate and repiration increasing, contractions in the colon also speed up and a rush to the toilet might be necessary. This can be very inconvenient to say the least but stress is a common factor in many gastrointestinal problems and should be considered before other more obscure diagnoses.

- Apart from cancer, sustained high levels of cortisol caused by ongoing stress often affects insulin and weight control. This can cause and/or exacerbate types 2 diabetes.

- Stress can affect blood pressure and increase the risk of heart problems.

- As well as causing these specific problems, stress can exacerbate almost all other problems and so it is important that we try to adopt a low stress lifestyle and adopt practices that reduce our stress levels whenever possible.

How to reduce Stress Hormones

There are many books that are devoted to this subject and so I can't possibly do this justice here. Most of the stress-reducing 'life practices' have come from Asia and involve meditation, 'being in the present' and practices that calm the mind and involve centreing.

These practices work very well for many people but I think that most of these are about not becoming stressed – which is extremely important – rather than reducing stress hormones if you are in an avoidable situation of intense stress.

Under a variety of stressful circumstances that might not in themsleves be preventable, you will feel anxious. You might be depressed. You are very likely to have digestive problems, impairment of your memory and concentration and you are unlikely to be able to sleep well. You might also get headaches and heart palpitations or develop a rash or a variety of other strange symptoms.

Having been in situations of intense stress where it was really unlikely that the stress could be resolved for some months at the earliest, I found a few different approaches helped me.

- The first approach is to evaluate your position and determine whether or not you can cope with it? Much of the stress we experience is caused by 'trying to hang on' in situations that are hopeless. What would happen if you just let go? Imagine you are standing on the side of a mountain and (fortunately) you have a parachute! Up till now, you have been fighting your problem by pushing against forces that you can't overcome. What would happen if – metaphorically speaking – you just opened your parachute and jumped? I think you will find that letting go is extremely empowering.

- Have at least one but preferably many nurturing massages. The massage will release most of your physical tension and if you have this in a salon that is burning aromotherapy oils, you will be greatly healed.

- Cry! Allow yourself to cry a great deal. Crying is very therapeutic. If you find it difficult to start crying about your problem you may find that watching a sad film allows you to let go. Don't be afraid to lie down and cry for many hours if your stress issue is very bad.

- Aerobic exercise usually helps you reduce tension. Don't overdo this at a time when your body is already highly stressed but a workout on a bike, running or rowing machine will usually help you.

- Finally, make sure that you develop a plan of action. There is little worse for your health than allowing yourself to be a victim so as soon as you have released some of the stress through one or more of the above actions, try to develop and initial plan immediately.

- Always be gentle with yourself through times of stress. You may have made some less than wise decisions that landed you in this bad place but being hard on yourself now will make things worse. Try to forgive yourself and focus on doing better in the next stage of your journey.

SLEEP – simple rules

Sleep, needed in huge amounts as a newborn and less as we gradually age, is a time of restoration of mind and body. All our physical systems are restored during sleep as well as our mood, memory and general brain function. Sleep has now been studied by large numbers of researchers internationally and there is still a great deal to learn. But the key message here is that good sleep is critical to your health and if you are having real problems you should seek help from a sleep clinic.

Everyone has some difficulties sleeping from time to time and as sleep is so important to your mental and physical health, here are a few simple reminders.

- Plan on having eight hours sleep each night and avoid too much stimulation in the last hour before bed. You should stop eating at least 2 hours before bed.

- Don't have the room lights too bright in the hour or so before bed – use lamps rather than central lights and **NEVER** turn on bright lights during the night. Have a torch or very low light bedside light that you can use if you need to move around during the night. Always sleep in a **dark room**. Make sure you block out any external lights that might shine into your room.

- Wear nothing or very light, non-restrictive clothing to bed.

- Don't overheat your bed. Use the coolest coverings that will keep you warm but never allow yourself to be hot. Unless you are in a very cold climate, don't heat your bedroom.

- In hot climates, try to cool yourself with ceiling fans (or similar) at night rather than air-conditioning where this is feasible. If the air is very humid you might benefit from a system that dries the air.

SUMMARY OF RECOMMENDATIONS TO REDUCE AGE-RELATED PROBLEMS AND ENHANCE HEALTH AND LONGEVITY

1. Eat fresh, local food whenever possible with a diverse range of ingredients to meet your nutritional needs. Retain the nutrients in your food by good storage and appropriate processing – make sure some of your daily intake is of raw food. Avoid ALL processed, smoked and cured foods. These should only ever be consumed in very low quantities.

2. Consume olive oil, sulfur-rich foods or a supplement such as MSM. Take GLA (Evening Primrose or equivalent) and consume vitamin K2 through Natto, Kimchi, cheese, yoghurt or (? other food). Make sure you have ample intake of other Vitamins and Minerals, especially A, D, E, B group and C plus essential minerals. If your food intake can't supply enough, take supplements. Beware of phytic acid as it depletes minerals. Try to make time to pre-soak grains and nuts but if so, make sure they are dried thoroughly.

3. Keep yourself and your skin well-hydrated. Drink high quality water throughout the day and protect your skin from sunburn.

4. Look after your teeth and make sure you chew. Twice daily brushing and flossing (or equivalent) is essential. Have regular dental check-ups.

5. Take care of your eyes and avoid too much glare. Have regular eye checks.

6. Avoid contagious illness and if you are ill, stay away from other people while you recover fully.

7. <u>Avoid</u> medications wherever possible (i.e. ask your doctor or health practitioner about the necessity of any drug) and understand all the ramifications of taking medications. <u>Avoid</u> over the counter pain killers whenever possible.

8. Exercise your **brain** and **body** using a diverse range of activities.

9. Avoid stress and take actions to reduce stress levels.

10. Don't overheat your home or yourself.

11. Check your plumbing and all other possible sources of chemical contaminants such as those used in the home for cleaning and/or pest control and fertilizers/herbicides used in the garden. Take care with all DYI activities!

12. Wear protective clothing whenever you might be exposed to chemicals and a face mask whenever you might be exposed to fumes. Use low toxicity products whenever they are a viable alternative.

13. **SLEEP WELL AND BE HAPPY**